WEIGHT LOSS

DIET COOKBOOK FOR BEGINNERS 2024

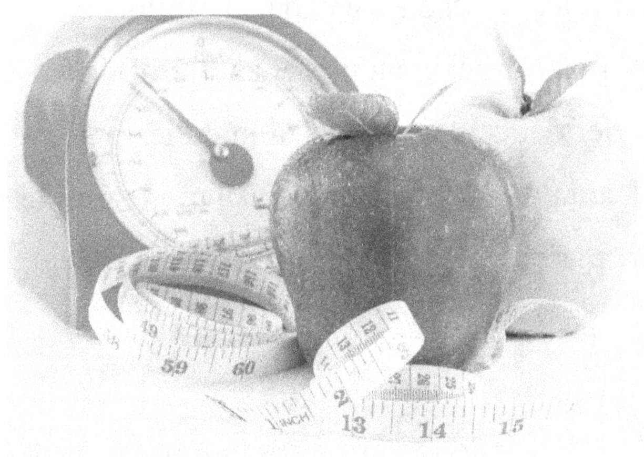

Eat Well, Live Well: A Journey to Weight Loss

Keri K. Huey

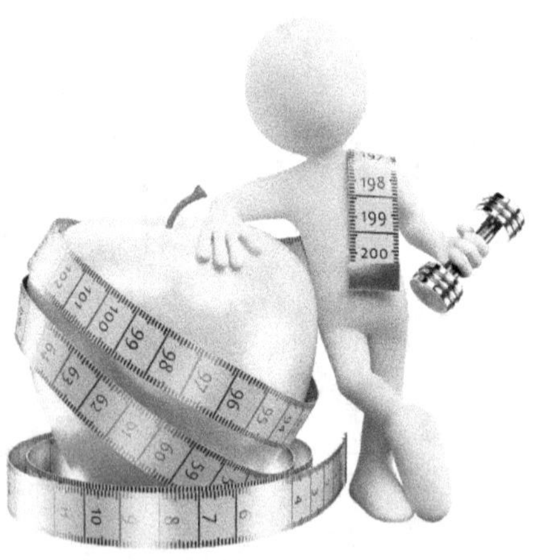

TABLE OF CONTENTS

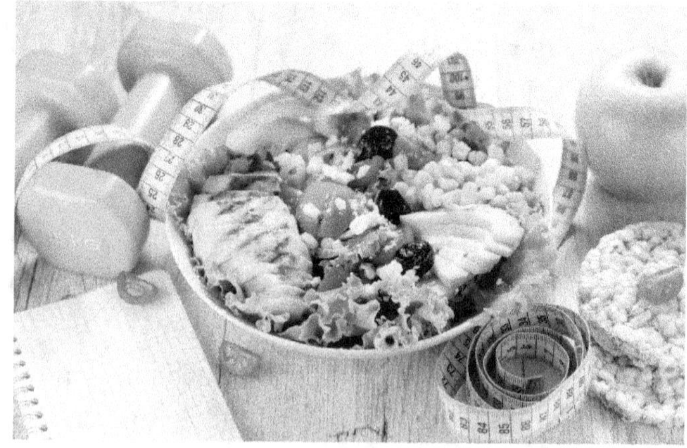

INTRODUCTION

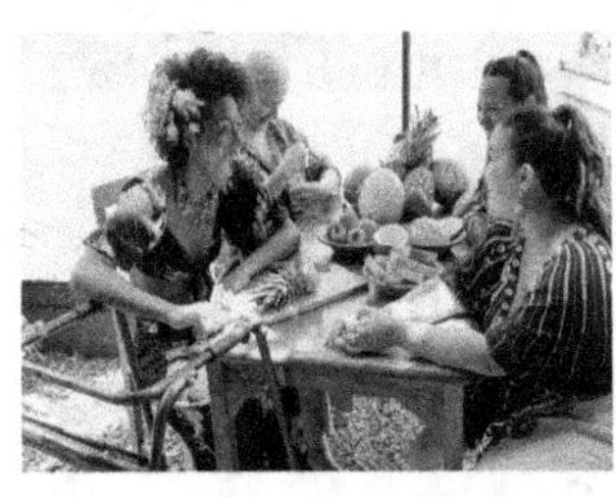 Once upon a time, there lived a group of inseparable friends known as the "Chubby Bunch." Charlie, Benny, Lisa, and Sarah were a lively quartet who shared a love for good food, laughter, and each other's company. However, their affection for culinary delights had taken a toll on their waistlines, and health concerns loomed over them like storm clouds.

One sunny day, as the friends gathered at their favorite local diner, a mysterious stranger named Professor NutriChef entered the scene. The eccentric professor, known for his brilliant culinary inventions, presented the Chubby Bunch with a revolutionary weight loss diet cookbook titled "Eat Well, Live Well."

Intrigued by the promise of shedding pounds without sacrificing flavor, the friends eagerly delved into the cookbook's pages. The recipes were a delightful fusion of vibrant colors, tantalizing aromas, and mouthwatering flavors. The Chubby Bunch decided to embark on a culinary adventure together, embracing the challenge of transforming their lifestyles.

Their journey began with a trip to the town's bustling farmers' market, where they excitedly picked fresh produce, lean proteins, and wholesome grains. Armed with shopping bags filled with healthy ingredients, they returned to Charlie's cozy kitchen, ready to create magic.

The Chubby Bunch navigated the recipes with enthusiasm, exchanging their favorite comfort foods for nutritious alternatives. Benny, the self-proclaimed barbecue king, discovered the joy of grilling lean meats and vegetables, while Lisa experimented with flavorful herb-infused dressings. Sarah, the dessert aficionado, mastered the art of crafting guilt-free sweets using natural sweeteners and innovative baking techniques.

As weeks passed, the aroma of healthy, delicious meals wafted through Harmonyville, drawing curious neighbors to the Chubby Bunch's gatherings. The friends not only shed excess weight but also gained a newfound energy that radiated positivity. Their transformation became an inspiration for the entire town.

The town of Harmonyville organized a grand festival to celebrate the Chubby Bunch's success and honor Professor NutriChef for his life-changing cookbook. The friends, once chubby and content, now stood proudly as ambassadors of health and happiness.

The story of the Chubby Bunch spread far and wide, capturing the attention of a publishing company. Encouraged by the townspeople, the friends collaborated to turn their culinary journey into a bestselling cookbook, spreading the message of the transformative power of healthy living.

And so, the Chubby Bunch's once-chubby lives evolved into a fabulous adventure of friendship, self-discovery, and the joy of savoring a life well-lived. The town of Harmonyville, once known for its love of hearty meals, became a beacon of health and happiness, all thanks to the magic of the

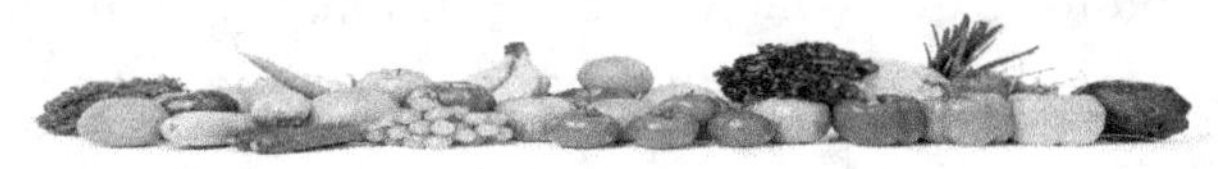

"Eat Well, Live Well" cookbook.

Welcome to Healthy Eating: A Journey to Weight Loss

Embarking on a journey to weight loss is more than a physical transformation; it's a profound exploration of self-discovery, resilience, and holistic well-being. As individuals set foot on this transformative path, they are greeted with the promise of a healthier, more vibrant life.

The journey begins with a shift in mindset, acknowledging that weight loss is not merely about shedding pounds but embracing a lifestyle centered around nourishing the body and mind. It involves cultivating mindfulness in eating, savoring each morsel, and developing a positive relationship with food.

Central to this expedition is the pursuit of a nutrient-rich plate, where fruits, vegetables, lean proteins, and whole grains become the building blocks of vitality. The journey encourages individuals to break free from sedentary habits, integrating enjoyable and sustainable physical activities into their daily routine.

In the kitchen, the journey unfolds as a culinary adventure, with individuals discovering the joy of cooking for wellness. Flavorful, wholesome meals become the cornerstone of this expedition, proving that healthy eating is not synonymous with deprivation but a celebration of diverse, satisfying, and nourishing food.

Yet, the journey to weight loss is not without its challenges. It requires perseverance, resilience, and a willingness to learn from both successes and setbacks. Through overcoming obstacles, individuals forge a path towards a healthier, more empowered version of themselves.

Ultimately, a journey to weight loss is an ongoing process of growth, self-love, and sustainable change. It is a testament to the incredible potential within each individual to transform their lives and embrace a future filled with vitality, balance, and the lasting rewards of a healthier lifestyle.

Understanding the Basics of Weight Loss Diets

Beginning a path toward a better living often entails navigating the vast terrain of weight reduction regimens. Understanding the foundations of different diets, each intended to satisfy particular requirements and tastes, is the key to success.

At the core of any effective weight loss diet is the principle of creating a caloric deficit. This means consuming fewer calories than the body expends, prompting it to burn stored fat for energy. While various diets employ different strategies, they all share the common goal of helping individuals shed excess weight.

One popular approach is the low-carbohydrate diet, emphasizing a reduction in the intake of sugars and starches. By minimizing these sources of rapid energy, the body turns to stored fat for fuel, leading to weight loss. The ketogenic diet takes this concept further by inducing a state of ketosis, where the body primarily burns fat for energy.

Conversely, the low-fat diet focuses on limiting dietary fats, promoting the consumption of lean proteins, whole grains, and fruits. This approach aims to reduce overall calorie intake while maintaining a balance of essential nutrients.

The Mediterranean diet, inspired by the traditional eating patterns of countries bordering the Mediterranean Sea, emphasizes whole foods, healthy fats, and a moderate intake of lean proteins. It is celebrated for not only aiding in weight loss but also promoting heart health.

Intermittent fasting has gained popularity as an eating pattern rather than a specific diet. It alternates between periods of eating and fasting, promoting fat loss by regulating insulin levels and enhancing metabolic flexibility.

Crucial to the success of any weight loss diet is sustainability and individualization. Understanding personal preferences, nutritional needs, and lifestyle factors ensures the chosen diet aligns with long-term goals. Additionally, incorporating regular physical activity and consulting with healthcare professionals contribute to a comprehensive and health-focused weight loss journey.

In navigating the world of weight loss diets, education and informed choices are the cornerstones of success. By grasping the basics and tailoring approaches to individual needs, individuals can embark on a journey towards sustainable weight loss and improved overall well-being.

Tips for Success on Your Weight Loss Journey

1. Set Realistic Goals: Define achievable, realistic, and time-bound goals. Break down larger objectives into smaller, manageable steps to celebrate progress along the way.

2. Embrace a Balanced Diet: Opt for nutrient-dense foods, including a variety of fruits, vegetables, lean proteins, and whole grains. Strive for balance and moderation, avoiding extreme diets for long-term sustainability.

3. Stay Hydrated: Drinking an adequate amount of water is crucial for overall health and can also aid in weight loss. Sometimes, feelings of hunger are actually signs of dehydration.

4. Practice Portion Control: Be mindful of portion sizes to avoid overeating. Use smaller plates, listen to your body's hunger cues, and savor each bite.

5. Incorporate Regular Exercise: Combine cardiovascular exercises, strength training, and flexibility exercises in your routine. Find activities you enjoy to make fitness a sustainable part of your lifestyle.

6. Get Adequate Sleep: Lack of sleep can negatively impact metabolism and increase cravings for unhealthy foods. Aim for 7-9 hours of quality sleep each night to support your weight loss efforts.

7. Track Your Progress: Keep a food journal, take regular measurements, or use apps to track your meals and physical activity. Monitoring your progress can provide valuable insights and keep you motivated.

8. Seek Support: Share your goals with friends, family, or join a supportive community. Having a support system can provide encouragement, accountability, and valuable advice.

9. Manage Stress: High stress levels can lead to emotional eating and hinder weight loss. Incorporate stress-management techniques such as meditation, yoga, or deep breathing exercises into your routine.

10. Celebrate Non-Scale Victories: Acknowledge and celebrate achievements beyond the scale, such as increased energy levels, improved mood, or better sleep. These positive changes are integral to your overall well-being.

11. Be Patient and Persistent: Sustainable weight loss takes time. Be patient with yourself, stay persistent, and view setbacks as opportunities to learn and readjust your approach.

12. Consult Professionals: Before making significant changes, consult with healthcare professionals, nutritionists, or fitness experts to ensure your weight loss plan is safe and tailored to your individual needs.

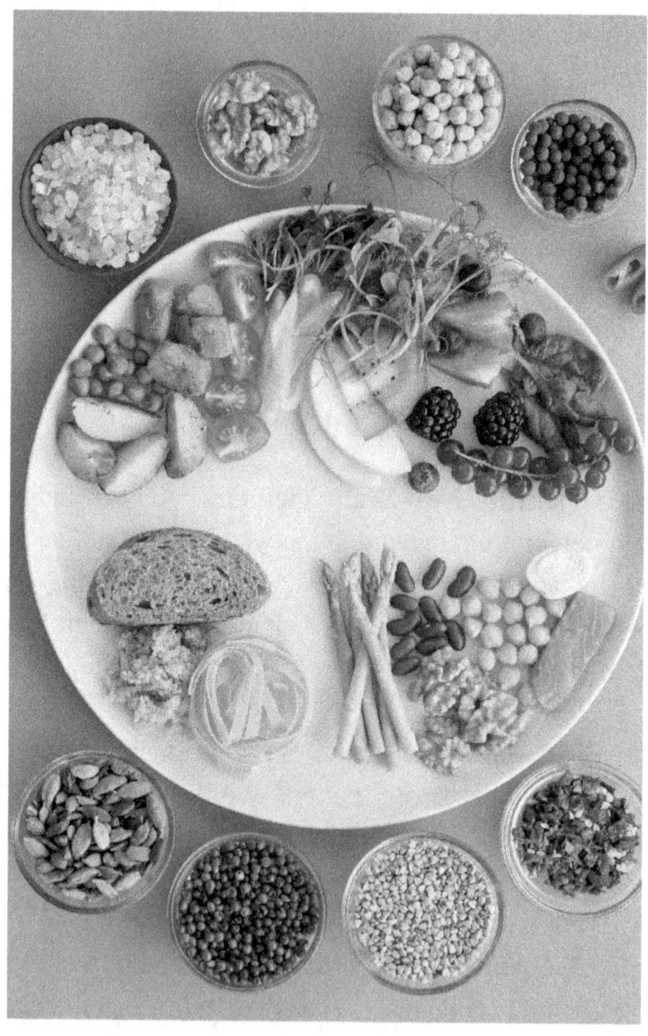

CHAPTER 1: NUTRITION FUNDAMENTALS

Understanding Macronutrients: Proteins, Carbohydrates, and Fats

Macronutrients, commonly referred to as macros, are essential components of our diet that provide the energy necessary for the body's functions and activities. Proteins, carbohydrates, and fats are the three primary macronutrients, each playing a unique role in maintaining optimal health.

Proteins:

- **Function**: Proteins are the building blocks of the body, crucial for the repair and growth of tissues. They also serve as enzymes, hormones, and antibodies, contributing to various physiological processes.

- **Sources:** Excellent sources of protein include lean meats, poultry, fish, eggs, dairy products, legumes, nuts, and seeds.

Carbohydrates:

- **Function:** Carbohydrates are the body's primary source of energy. They provide glucose, which fuels brain function and supports physical activities. Carbohydrates also assist in regulating blood sugar levels.

- **Sources:** Healthy carbohydrate sources include whole grains, fruits, vegetables, legumes, and dairy products. Opt for complex carbohydrates for sustained energy release.

Fats:

- **Function:** Fats are essential for the absorption of fat-soluble vitamins (A, D, E, K), brain function, and the production of hormones. They also provide a concentrated source of energy.

- **Sources:** Healthy fat sources include avocados, nuts, seeds, olive oil, fatty fish (like salmon and mackerel), and plant-based oils. Limit saturated and trans fats found in processed and fried foods.

Understanding how to balance these macronutrients is crucial for a well-rounded and nutritious diet. The proportion of each macronutrient can vary based on individual goals, health conditions, and lifestyle. For example, athletes may require a higher protein intake for muscle repair, while individuals aiming for weight loss might focus on a balanced combination of all three macronutrients.

It's important to note that a balanced diet involves not only the right proportions of macronutrients but also a variety of micronutrients (vitamins and minerals). Consulting with a healthcare professional or a registered dietitian can help tailor your diet to meet your specific needs, ensuring optimal health and well-being.

Micronutrients and Their Role in Weight Loss

While macronutrients (proteins, carbohydrates, and fats) are crucial for providing energy, micronutrients play a vital role in supporting various physiological functions and can contribute to a successful weight loss journey. Micronutrients include essential vitamins and minerals, each with specific functions that aid overall health and well-being.

Vitamins:

- **Vitamin A:** Supports vision, immune function, and skin health. Found in sweet potatoes, carrots, spinach, and dairy products.
- *Vitamin D:* Essential for bone health and can influence weight loss. Sources include sunlight exposure, fatty fish, and fortified dairy products.

- **Vitamin C:** Aids in collagen synthesis and enhances iron absorption. Found in citrus fruits, strawberries, bell peppers, and broccoli.

- **B Vitamins (B1, B2, B3, B6, B12):** Contribute to energy metabolism, neurological function, and red blood cell production. Sources include whole grains, lean meats, dairy products, and leafy greens.

Minerals:

- **Calcium:** Supports bone health and may play a role in fat metabolism. Found in dairy products, leafy greens, and fortified plant-based milk.

- **Iron:** Essential for oxygen transport in the blood. Sources include lean meats, legumes, spinach, and fortified cereals.

- **Magnesium:** Aids in energy production and muscle function. Found in nuts, seeds, whole grains, and leafy greens.

- **Zinc:** Supports immune function and plays a role in metabolism. Sources include meat, dairy, nuts, and legumes.

Role of Micronutrients in Weight Loss:

1. Metabolism Support: Micronutrients, such as B vitamins and magnesium, play a crucial role in energy metabolism, helping the body convert food into usable energy. A well-functioning metabolism contributes to effective weight management.

2. Appetite Regulation: Some micronutrients, like vitamin D and calcium, may influence appetite regulation. Ensuring an adequate intake of these nutrients can contribute to better appetite control and, consequently, weight loss.

3. Nutrient Absorption: Micronutrients support the absorption of macronutrients, ensuring that the body efficiently utilizes the energy derived from proteins, carbohydrates, and fats.

4. Energy Production: Micronutrients contribute to the production of energy at the cellular level, promoting overall vitality and supporting physical activity, an essential component of weight loss.

Portion Control and Mindful Eating

In the quest for a healthy and balanced lifestyle, two key practices stand out: portion control and mindful eating. These habits not only contribute to weight management but also foster a positive relationship with food, allowing individuals to savor each bite and make conscious choices about what and how much they consume.

Portion Control:

Portion control involves managing the amount of food served during meals and snacks. It is a fundamental aspect of maintaining a balanced diet and preventing overeating. Here are some tips to incorporate portion control into your eating habits:

1. Use Smaller Plates: Opt for smaller plates and bowls to create the illusion of a fuller plate, promoting satisfaction with smaller portions.

2. Divide Your Plate: Visualize your plate divided into sections: half for vegetables, a quarter for lean protein, and a quarter for carbohydrates. This simple guideline encourages a balanced and portioned meal.

3. Be Mindful of Liquid Calories: Watch your intake of caloric beverages, as they can contribute significantly to overall energy consumption. Choose water, herbal tea, or other low-calorie options.

4. Listen to Your Body: Pay attention to hunger and fullness cues. Eat slowly and stop when you feel satisfied, not overly full. This allows your body to register satiety effectively.

5. Avoid Distractions: Minimize distractions, such as watching TV or working on your computer, while eating. Focus on the sensory experience of eating to recognize feelings of fullness.

Mindful Eating:

Mindful eating involves being fully present and attentive during meals, savoring flavors, textures, and the overall experience of eating. Here are tips to cultivate mindful eating habits:

1. Eat Without Distractions: Turn off electronic devices, put away books, and create a dedicated space for meals. This allows you to focus on the act of eating and the sensory experience of each bite.

2. Chew Thoroughly: Take the time to chew your food slowly and thoroughly. This not only aids digestion but also allows your brain to register fullness more effectively.

3. Engage Your Senses: Appreciate the colors, aromas, and textures of your food. Engaging your senses enhances the enjoyment of your meals and fosters a mindful approach to eating.

4. Pause Between Bites: Put your utensils down between bites. This simple practice encourages a slower eating pace and enables you to recognize when you're satisfied.

5. Check in with Hunger Levels: Before reaching for seconds, assess your hunger levels. Are you eating out of habit or true hunger? Mindful eating involves tuning into your body's signals.

By combining portion control with mindful eating, individuals can develop a sustainable and balanced approach to nutrition. These practices not only contribute to weight management but also promote a healthier relationship with food, emphasizing quality, enjoyment, and awareness.

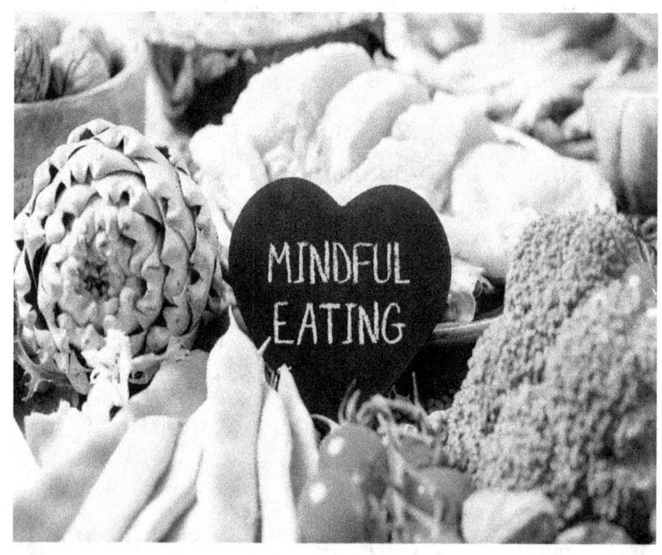

CHAPTER 2: SETTING UP YOUR KITCHEN

Essential Kitchen Tools for Healthy Cooking

Equipping your kitchen with the right tools is a fundamental step in embracing a healthy cooking lifestyle. These essential kitchen tools not only make meal preparation more efficient but also contribute to the creation of nutritious and delicious dishes:

1. **High-Quality Knife Set:**

A sharp, reliable knife set is the cornerstone of any well-equipped kitchen. Invest in a variety of knives, including a chef's knife, paring knife, and serrated knife, to handle different cutting tasks with precision.

2. **Cutting Boards:**

Choose durable, easy-to-clean cutting boards made of materials like bamboo or plastic. Having separate boards for meat, vegetables, and fruits helps prevent cross-contamination.

3. **Non-Stick Cookware:**

Non-stick pans and pots reduce the need for excessive oil when cooking. Opt for high-quality, non-toxic non-stick cookware to prepare meals with minimal added fats.

4. Steamer Basket:

A steamer basket is a versatile tool for cooking vegetables, seafood, and even dumplings. Steaming preserves nutrients, and this method requires little to no added oil.

5. Food Processor or Blender:

These appliances are indispensable for preparing smoothies, soups, sauces, and homemade dips. They make it easy to incorporate nutritious ingredients like fruits, vegetables, and nuts into your diet.

6. Measuring Tools:

Precise measurements are crucial for maintaining portion control and accurately following recipes. Invest in measuring cups and spoons to ensure you're using the right amounts of ingredients.

7. Digital Food Scale:

A digital food scale is an excellent tool for tracking portions and managing calorie intake. It's particularly helpful when portioning proteins, grains, and other ingredients for balanced meals.

8. Vegetable Spiralizer:

For a creative and healthy twist to your meals, a vegetable spiralizer allows you to transform vegetables like zucchini and sweet potatoes into noodle-like strands. It's a fantastic alternative to traditional pasta.

9. Oven Thermometer:

Achieving accurate temperatures in your oven is essential for perfectly cooked, healthy meals. An oven thermometer ensures that your recipes are cooked to perfection without excessive use of oils or fats.

10. Storage Containers:

Having a variety of storage containers helps you organize and store prepped ingredients and leftovers. Opt for glass containers for reheating and reducing exposure to harmful chemicals found in some plastics.

Equipping your kitchen with these essential tools sets the stage for a seamless and enjoyable healthy cooking experience. As you prioritize nutrient-rich ingredients and mindful preparation, these tools will become invaluable allies in your journey toward maintaining a wholesome and balanced diet.

Stocking Your Pantry for Success

Stocking your pantry for success is a pivotal step in fostering a nutritious and sustainable approach to cooking. A well-stocked pantry not only streamlines meal preparation but also ensures you have the essential ingredients to create healthy, flavorful dishes. Here's a guide to building a pantry that supports your wellness goals:

1. Whole Grains: Opt for staples like brown rice, quinoa, oats, and whole-grain pasta. These complex carbohydrates provide sustained energy and are rich in fiber.

2. Canned Legumes: Beans, lentils, and chickpeas are excellent sources of plant-based protein and fiber. Keep a variety of canned legumes for quick and convenient meal additions.

3. Healthy Oils: Choose heart-healthy oils such as olive oil, avocado oil, or coconut oil. These fats add flavor and nutritional value to your dishes.

3. Nuts and Seeds: Almonds, walnuts, chia seeds, and flaxseeds are nutrient-dense additions to your pantry, providing essential omega-3 fatty acids and a satisfying crunch.

4. Herbs and Spices: Build a diverse collection of herbs and spices to enhance the flavor of your meals without relying on excessive salt or sugar. Consider staples like garlic powder, cumin, turmeric, and dried herbs.

5. Canned Tomatoes: A versatile ingredient, canned tomatoes serve as a base for sauces, soups, and stews. Look for options without added sugars or preservatives.

6. Low-Sodium Broth: Keep vegetable, chicken, or bone broth on hand for creating flavorful bases for soups and stews.

7. Whole Food Sweeteners: Opt for natural sweeteners like honey, maple syrup, or agave nectar to satisfy your sweet tooth while avoiding refined sugars.

8. Whole Grain Flour: For baking, choose whole grain flours such as whole wheat or almond flour for a healthier twist.

9. Dried Fruits: Unsweetened dried fruits like raisins, apricots, or cranberries can add natural sweetness to recipes and snacks.

Regularly assess and replenish your pantry to avoid running out of key ingredients. With a well-stocked pantry, you'll have the foundation for creating wholesome, delicious meals that align with your health and wellness objectives. Planning and organizing your pantry not only simplify your cooking routine but also empower you to make nutritious choices effortlessly.

Smart Grocery Shopping Tips and Meal Planning

Efficient grocery shopping and strategic meal planning are essential components of maintaining a healthy and balanced lifestyle. Here's a guide to help you navigate the aisles and plan meals that align with your wellness goals:

1. Make a List:

- Plan your meals for the week and create a detailed shopping list. This reduces the likelihood of impulse purchases and helps you stay focused on your nutritional needs.

2. **Shop the Perimeter:**
   - The perimeter of the grocery store often houses fresh produce, lean proteins, and dairy. Focus on these areas to incorporate nutrient-dense, whole foods into your diet.

3. **Read Labels:**
   - Be mindful of ingredient lists and nutritional labels. Choose items with minimal additives, lower sodium content, and limited added sugars.

4. **Buy in Bulk:**
   - Purchase non-perishable items like grains, legumes, and nuts in bulk. This not only reduces packaging waste but can also be more cost-effective.

5. **Choose Seasonal Produce:**
   - Opt for fruits and vegetables that are in season. They tend to be fresher, more flavorful, and may be more budget-friendly.

6. **Stick to a Schedule:**
   - Choose a time for grocery shopping when you're not rushed. This allows you to make thoughtful choices and avoid last-minute decisions.

7. **Explore the Frozen Section:**
   - Stock up on frozen fruits, vegetables, and proteins. They have a longer shelf life and

are just as nutritious as their fresh counterparts.

8. Limit Processed Foods:

- Minimize purchases of highly processed and packaged foods. Instead, focus on whole, minimally processed options to enhance the nutritional quality of your meals.

Meal Planning:

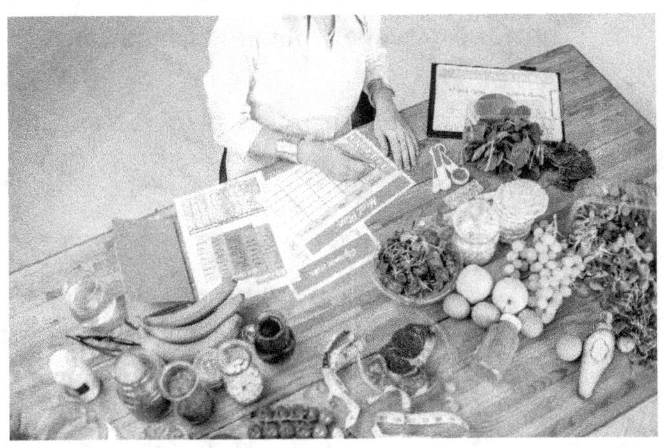

1. Batch Cooking:

- Prepare large batches of staples like grains, proteins, and vegetables over the weekend. Use these as building blocks for various meals throughout the week.

2. Plan for Leftovers:

- Design meals that can yield leftovers for the next day's lunch or dinner. This saves time and ensures you have nutritious options readily available.

3. **Balance Macronutrients:**
   - Aim for a balance of proteins, carbohydrates, and healthy fats in each meal. This promotes satiety and provides a well-rounded nutritional profile.

4. **Include a Variety of Colors:**
   - Incorporate a diverse range of fruits and vegetables with different colors to ensure a broad spectrum of vitamins and minerals.

5. **Snack Smart:**
   - Plan for healthy snacks to avoid reaching for less nutritious options when hunger strikes between meals.

6. **Be Flexible:**
   - Stay flexible with your meal plan. Life can be unpredictable, and having alternatives allows you to adapt without compromising your nutritional goals.

By combining smart grocery shopping with thoughtful meal planning, you set the stage for a week of nourishing and satisfying meals. This approach not only supports your health and wellness but also saves time and reduces food waste.

CHAPTER 3: BREAKFASTS TO KICKSTART YOUR DAY

Energizing Smoothie Bowls and Breakfast Parfaits Recipes

Recipe 1: Berry Blast Smoothie Bowl

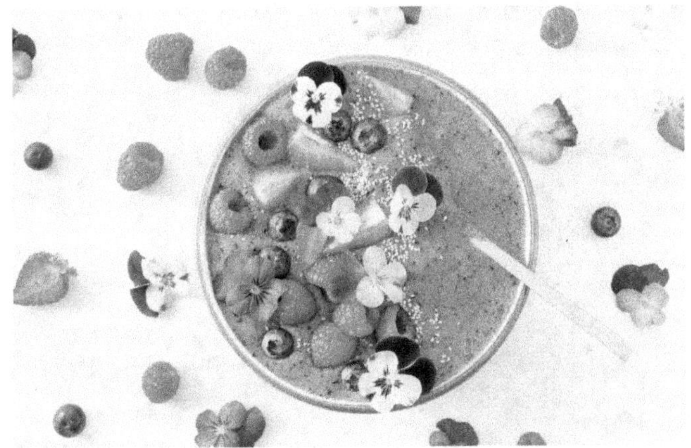

Ingredients:

- 1 cup mixed berries (strawberries, blueberries, raspberries)
- 1 frozen banana
- 1/2 cup Greek yogurt
- 1/4 cup almond milk
- 1 tablespoon chia seeds
- Toppings: granola, sliced strawberries, coconut flakes

Instructions:

1. Blend mixed berries, frozen banana, Greek yogurt, almond milk, and chia seeds until smooth.
2. Pour the smoothie into a bowl.
3. Top with granola, sliced strawberries, and coconut flakes.
4. Enjoy immediately.

Nutrition Information:

- Calories: 350
- Protein: 15g
- Fat: 10g
- Carbohydrates: 50g
- Fiber: 12g
- Prep Time: 5 minutes
- Serves: 1

Recipe 2: Tropical Paradise Breakfast Parfait

Ingredients:

- 1 cup pineapple chunks
- 1/2 cup mango chunks
- 1/2 cup vanilla Greek yogurt
- 1/4 cup granola
- 1 tablespoon shredded coconut
- Drizzle of honey

Instructions:

1. Layer pineapple chunks at the bottom of a glass or jar.
2. Add a layer of mango chunks on top.
3. Spoon vanilla Greek yogurt over the fruit.
4. Sprinkle granola and shredded coconut on top.
5. Drizzle with honey.
6. Repeat the layers.
7. Finish with a drizzle of honey on the top layer.
8. Refrigerate for at least 30 minutes before serving.

Nutrition Information:
- Calories: 400
- Protein: 15g
- Fat: 8g
- Carbohydrates: 70g
- Fiber: 6g
- Prep Time: 10 minutes
- Serves: 2

Recipe 3: Green Goddess Smoothie Bowl

Ingredients:
- 1 cup spinach leaves
- 1/2 avocado
- 1/2 banana
- 1/2 cup plain Greek yogurt
- 1/4 cup almond milk
- Toppings: sliced kiwi, hemp seeds, sliced almonds

Instructions:

1. Blend spinach, avocado, banana, Greek yogurt, and almond milk until smooth.
2. Pour into a bowl.
3. Top with sliced kiwi, hemp seeds, and sliced almonds.
4. Enjoy this nutrient-packed bowl.

Nutrition Information:

- Calories: 320
- Protein: 15g
- Fat: 18g
- Carbohydrates: 30g
- Fiber: 9g
- Prep Time: 5 minutes
- Serves: 1

Recipe 4: Apple Cinnamon Breakfast Parfait

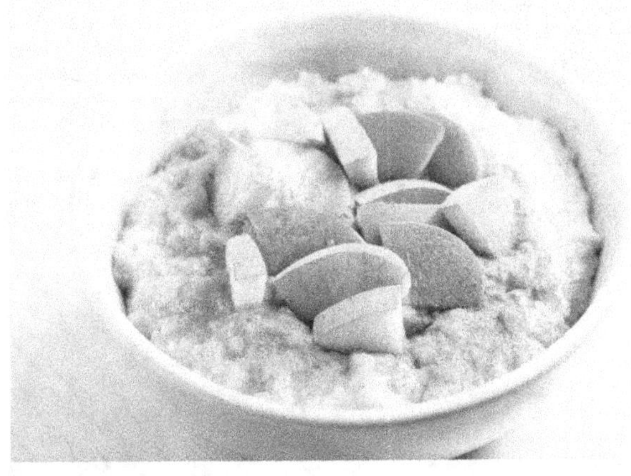

Ingredients:

- 1 cup diced apples
- 1/2 cup vanilla yogurt
- 1/4 cup granola
- 1 tablespoon chopped walnuts
- Sprinkle of cinnamon

Instructions:

1. In a glass or jar, layer diced apples at the bottom.
2. Spoon vanilla yogurt over the apples.
3. Sprinkle granola and chopped walnuts on top.
4. Repeat the layers.
5. Finish with a sprinkle of cinnamon.
6. Refrigerate for at least 30 minutes before serving.

Nutrition Information:

- Calories: 320
- Protein: 8g
- Fat: 12g
- Carbohydrates: 45g
- Fiber: 7g
- Prep Time: 10 minutes
- -Serves: 2

Recipe 5: Chocolate Peanut Butter Smoothie Bowl

Ingredients:

- 1 frozen banana
- 2 tablespoons peanut butter
- 1 tablespoon cocoa powder
- 1/2 cup chocolate protein powder
- 1/2 cup almond milk
- Toppings: sliced bananas, crushed peanuts, dark chocolate shavings

Instructions:

1. Blend frozen banana, peanut butter, cocoa powder, chocolate protein powder, and almond milk until smooth.
2. Pour into a bowl.

3. Top with sliced bananas, crushed peanuts, and dark chocolate shavings.

4. Dive into this indulgent yet healthy treat.

Nutrition Information:
- Calories: 420
- Protein: 25g
- Fat: 18g
- Carbohydrates: 45g
- Fiber: 8g
- Prep Time: 5 minutes
- Serves: 1

Recipe 6: Mixed Berry Yogurt Parfait

Ingredients:
- 1 cup mixed berries (strawberries, blueberries, raspberries)
- 1 cup vanilla Greek yogurt
- 1/4 cup granola
- Drizzle of honey
- Fresh mint leaves for garnish

Instructions:
1. In a glass, layer mixed berries.
2. Spoon vanilla Greek yogurt over the berries.
3. Sprinkle granola on top.
4. Repeat the layers.
5. Finish with a drizzle of honey and garnish with fresh mint leaves.

6. Refrigerate for at least 30 minutes before serving.

Nutrition Information:
- Calories: 280
- Protein: 15g
- Fat: 5g
- Carbohydrates: 45g
- Fiber: 6g
- Prep Time: 10 minutes
- Serves: 2

Wholesome Oatmeal and Quinoa Breakfast Recipes

Recipe 1: Classic Maple Cinnamon Oatmeal

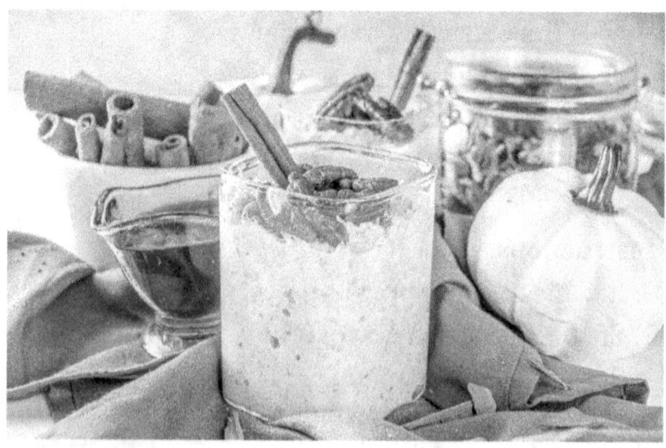

Ingredients:

- 1 cup rolled oats
- 2 cups water or milk
- 1 tablespoon maple syrup
- 1/2 teaspoon cinnamon
- Fresh berries for topping

Instructions:

1. In a saucepan, bring water or milk to a boil.
2. Stir in rolled oats, reduce heat, and simmer for 5-7 minutes, stirring occasionally.
3. Once oats are cooked, remove from heat and stir in maple syrup and cinnamon.
4. Top with fresh berries.
5. Enjoy your warm and comforting maple cinnamon oatmeal.

Nutrition Information:

- Calories: 300
- Protein: 10g
- Fat: 5g
- Carbohydrates: 55g
- Fiber: 8g
- Prep Time: 2 minutes
- Cook Time: 7 minutes
- Serves: 2

Recipe 2: Quinoa Breakfast Bowl

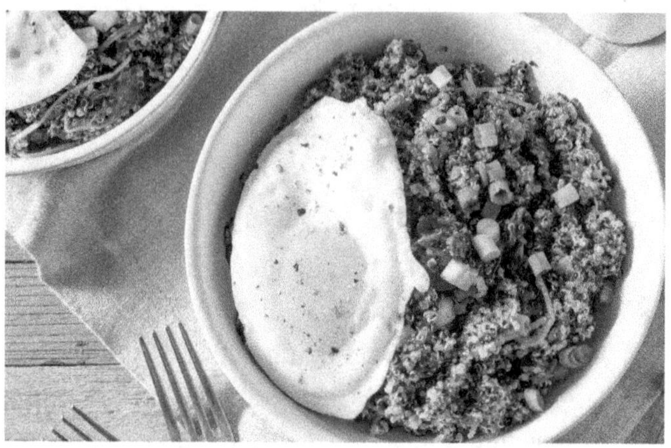

Ingredients:

- 1 cup cooked quinoa
- 1/2 cup almond milk
- 1 tablespoon honey
- 1/4 cup chopped nuts (e.g., almonds, walnuts)
- Sliced banana for topping

Instructions:

1. In a bowl, combine cooked quinoa, almond milk, honey, and chopped nuts.
2. Stir well to combine.
3. Top with sliced banana.
4. Serve this protein-packed quinoa breakfast bowl warm.

Nutrition Information:

- Calories: 320
- Protein: 12g
- Fat: 10g
- Carbohydrates: 50g
- Fiber: 6g
- Prep Time: 5 minutes
- Cook Time: 15 minutes (for quinoa)
- Serves: 2

Recipe 3: Apple Cinnamon Oatmeal

Ingredients:
- 1 cup steel-cut oats
- 2 cups water or milk
- 1 apple, diced
- 1/2 teaspoon cinnamon
- 1 tablespoon almond butter
- Chopped nuts for topping

Instructions:
1. In a pot, combine steel-cut oats, water or milk, diced apple, and cinnamon.
2. Bring to a boil, then reduce heat and simmer for 20-25 minutes, stirring occasionally.
3. Once cooked, stir in almond butter.
4. Top with chopped nuts.
5. Enjoy this warm and flavorful apple cinnamon oatmeal.

Nutrition Information:

- Calories: 350
- Protein: 10g
- Fat: 10g
- Carbohydrates: 55g
- Fiber: 8g
- Prep Time: 5 minutes
- Cook Time: 25 minutes
- Serves: 2

Recipe 4: Berry Quinoa Parfait

Ingredients:
- 1 cup cooked quinoa
- 1/2 cup Greek yogurt
- 1 cup mixed berries (strawberries, blueberries, raspberries)
- 1 tablespoon honey
- Granola for topping

Instructions:
1. In a glass or bowl, layer cooked quinoa, Greek yogurt, and mixed berries.
2. Drizzle honey over the layers.
3. Repeat the layers.
4. Top with granola for added crunch.
5. Serve this wholesome berry quinoa parfait chilled.

Nutrition Information:
- Calories: 320

- Protein: 15g
- Fat: 8g
- Carbohydrates: 50g
- Fiber: 8g
- Prep Time: 10 minutes
- Cook Time: 15 minutes (for quinoa)
- Serves: 2

Recipe 5: Peanut Butter Banana Oatmeal

Ingredients:
- 1 cup old-fashioned oats
- 2 cups water or milk
- 2 tablespoons peanut butter
- 1 banana, sliced
- 1 tablespoon chia seeds

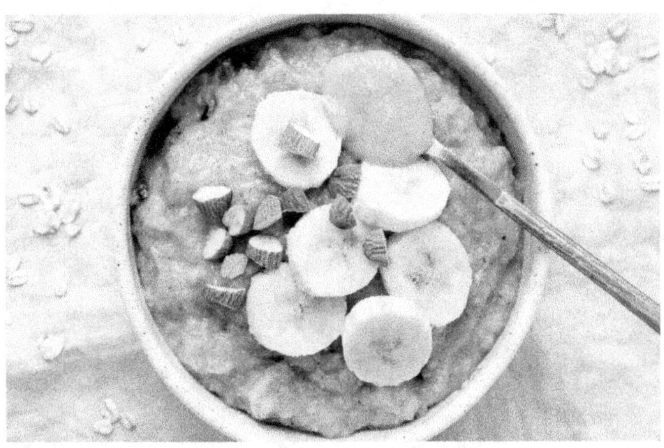

Instructions:
1. In a saucepan, bring water or milk to a boil.

2. Stir in old-fashioned oats and cook for 5-7 minutes, stirring occasionally.
3. Once oats are cooked, stir in peanut butter.
4. Top with sliced banana and chia seeds.
5. Enjoy this protein-packed peanut butter banana oatmeal.

Nutrition Information:
- Calories: 380
- Protein: 15g
- Fat: 15g
- Carbohydrates: 50g
- Fiber: 9g
- Prep Time: 2 minutes
- Cook Time: 7 minutes
- Serves: 2

Protein-Packed Breakfasts for Sustained Energy

Recipe 1: Veggie and Egg Breakfast Wrap

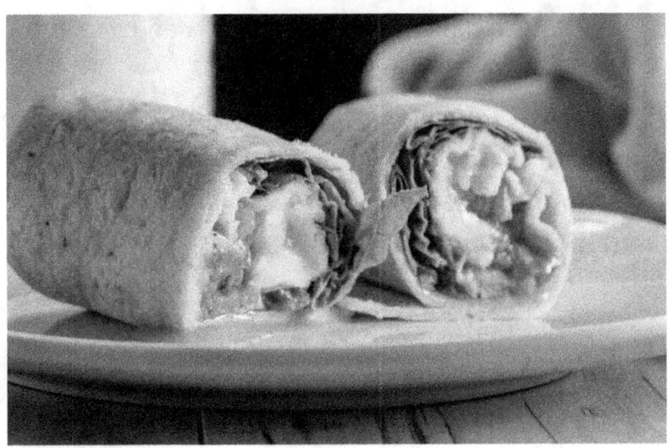

Ingredients:

- 2 whole eggs, beaten
- 1/4 cup diced bell peppers
- 1/4 cup diced tomatoes
- 2 tablespoons diced red onion
- 1/4 cup shredded cheese
- 1 whole wheat tortilla
- Salt and pepper to taste
- Fresh cilantro for garnish (optional)

Instructions:

1. In a non-stick pan over medium heat, sauté bell peppers, tomatoes, and red onion until softened.

2. Pour beaten eggs into the pan, stirring to combine with the vegetables.
3. Add shredded cheese and continue stirring until eggs are cooked through.
4. Season with salt and pepper.
5. Warm the whole wheat tortilla and spoon the egg mixture onto it.
6. Roll into a wrap, garnish with fresh cilantro if desired, and serve.

Nutrition Information:
- Calories: 350
- Protein: 23g
- Fat: 18g
- Carbohydrates: 26g
- Fiber: 4g
- Prep Time: 10 minutes
- Cook Time: 5 minutes
- Serves: 1

Recipe 2: Greek Yogurt Parfait with strawberry

Ingredients:
- 1 cup Greek yogurt (unsweetened)
- 1/2 cup mixed berries (strawberries, blueberries, raspberries)
- 2 tablespoons honey
- 1/4 cup granola

- 1 tablespoon chia seeds

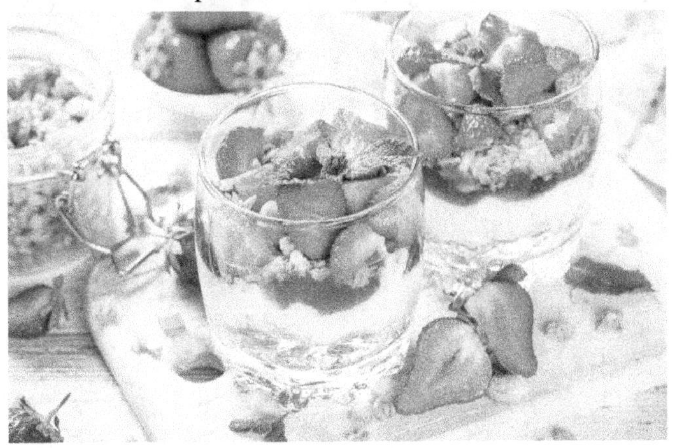

Instructions:

1. In a glass or bowl, layer Greek yogurt.
2. Add a layer of mixed berries.
3. Drizzle honey over the berries.
4. Sprinkle granola and chia seeds on top.
5. Repeat the layers.
6. Refrigerate for at least 30 minutes before serving.

Nutrition Information:

- Calories: 400
- Protein: 25g
- Fat: 12g
- Carbohydrates: 55g
- Fiber: 8g
- Prep Time: 5 minutes
- Serves: 1

Recipe 3: Quinoa and Spinach Breakfast Bowl

Ingredients:

- 1/2 cup cooked quinoa
- 1 cup fresh spinach
- 1/4 cup diced cherry tomatoes
- 1/4 cup feta cheese, crumbled
- 1 poached egg
- 1 tablespoon olive oil
- Salt and pepper to taste

Instructions:

1. In a pan, sauté fresh spinach in olive oil until wilted.
2. In a bowl, layer cooked quinoa.
3. Add sautéed spinach, diced cherry tomatoes, and crumbled feta cheese.
4. Top with a poached egg.
5. Season with salt and pepper.
6. Drizzle with additional olive oil if desired and serve.

Nutrition Information:

- Calories: 380
- Protein: 18g
- Fat: 20g
- Carbohydrates: 30g
- Fiber: 5g

- Prep Time: 15 minutes
- Cook Time: 10 minutes
- Serves: 1

Recipe 4: Peanut Butter Banana Protein Smoothie

Ingredients:
- 1 banana
- 1 scoop vanilla protein powder
- 1 tablespoon peanut butter
- 1 cup almond milk
- 1/2 cup ice cubes

Instructions:
1. In a blender, combine banana, vanilla protein powder, peanut butter, almond milk, and ice cubes.
2. Blend until smooth and creamy.
3. Pour into a glass and enjoy immediately.

Nutrition Information:
- Calories: 380
- Protein: 30g
- Fat: 15g
- Carbohydrates: 35g
- Fiber: 6g
- Prep Time: 5 minutes
- Serves: 1

CHAPTER 4: SATISFYING LUNCHES AND QUICK SNACKS

Fresh and Flavorful Salad Creations

Recipe 1: Summer Citrus Salad

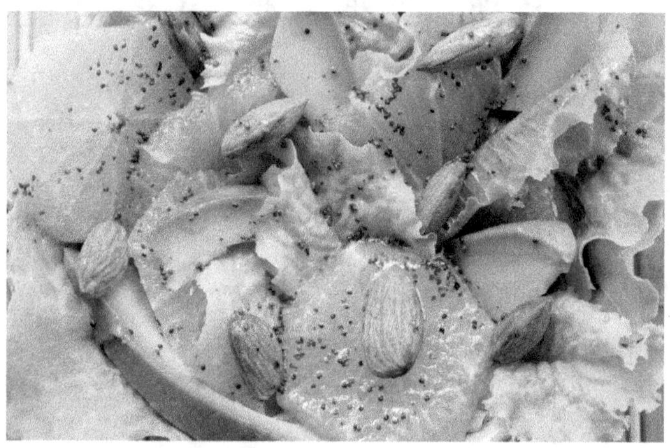

Ingredients:
- 4 cups mixed greens (arugula, spinach, and watercress)
- 1 orange, segmented
- 1 grapefruit, segmented
- 1/2 cup cherry tomatoes, halved
- 1/4 cup feta cheese, crumbled
- 2 tablespoons balsamic vinaigrette

- Salt and pepper to taste

Instructions:

1. In a large bowl, combine mixed greens, orange segments, grapefruit segments, cherry tomatoes, and feta cheese.
2. Drizzle with balsamic vinaigrette.
3. Toss gently to combine.
4. Season with salt and pepper to taste.
5. Serve immediately.

Nutrition Information:

- Calories: 200
- Protein: 5g
- Fat: 10g
- Carbohydrates: 25g
- Fiber: 6g
- Prep Time: 10 minutes
- Serves: 2

Recipe 2: Quinoa and Avocado Power Salad

Ingredients:

- 1 cup cooked quinoa, cooled
- 1 cup cherry tomatoes, halved
- 1 cucumber, diced
- 1 avocado, sliced
- 1/4 cup red onion, finely chopped

- 2 tablespoons olive oil
- 1 tablespoon lemon juice
- Fresh basil leaves for garnish
- Salt and pepper to taste

Instructions:

1. In a large bowl, combine quinoa, cherry tomatoes, cucumber, avocado, and red onion.
2. In a small bowl, whisk together olive oil and lemon juice to make the dressing.
3. Drizzle the dressing over the salad and toss gently.
4. Garnish with fresh basil leaves.
5. Season with salt and pepper to taste.
6. Serve chilled.

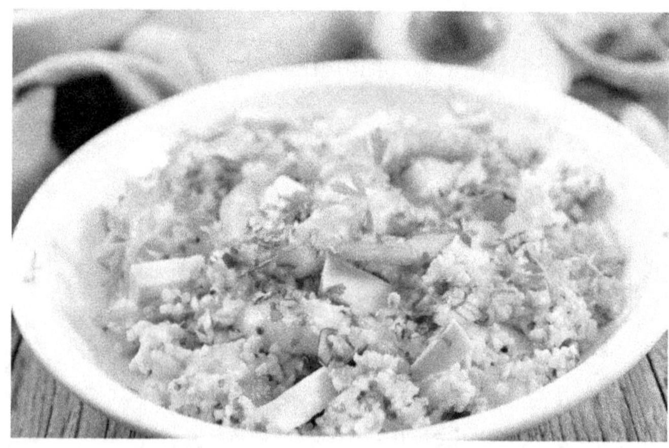

Nutrition Information:

- Calories: 320
- Protein: 8g

- Fat: 18g
- Carbohydrates: 35g
- Fiber: 7g
- Prep Time: 15 minutes
- Serves: 2

Recipe 3: Grilled Chicken and Mango Tango Salad

Ingredients:
- 2 boneless, skinless chicken breasts, grilled and sliced
- 2 cups mixed salad greens
- 1 mango, peeled and diced
- 1/4 cup red bell pepper, diced
- 1/4 cup red onion, thinly sliced
- 2 tablespoons lime juice
- 1 tablespoon honey
- 1 tablespoon cilantro, chopped
- Salt and pepper to taste

Instructions:
1. In a large bowl, combine grilled chicken, mixed salad greens, mango, red bell pepper, and red onion.
2. In a small bowl, whisk together lime juice, honey, and cilantro to make the dressing.
3. Drizzle the dressing over the salad and toss gently.

4. Season with salt and pepper to taste.
5. Serve immediately.

Nutrition Information:
- Calories: 300
- Protein: 25g
- Fat: 8g
- Carbohydrates: 30g
- Fiber: 5g
- Prep Time: 20 minutes
- Cook Time: 15 minutes
- Serves: 2

Recipe 4: Caprese Salad with a Twist

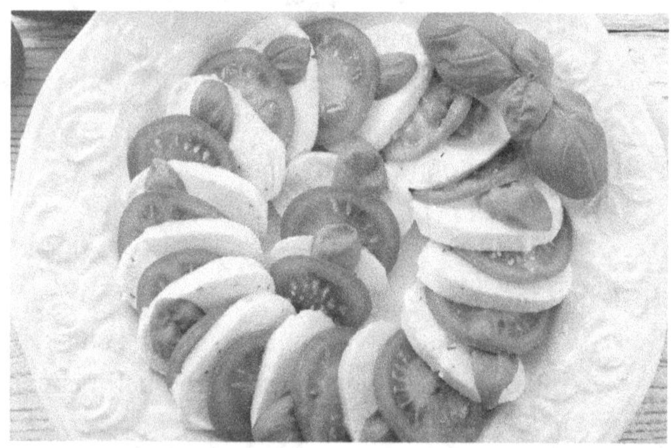

Ingredients:
- 2 cups cherry tomatoes, halved
- 1 cup fresh mozzarella balls
- 1 cup fresh basil leaves

- 2 tablespoons balsamic glaze
- 2 tablespoons extra virgin olive oil
- Salt and pepper to taste

Instructions:

1. In a large bowl, combine cherry tomatoes, fresh mozzarella balls, and fresh basil leaves.
2. Drizzle with balsamic glaze and extra virgin olive oil.
3. Toss gently to combine.
4. Season with salt and pepper to taste.
5. Serve chilled.

Nutrition Information:

- Calories: 250
- Protein: 12g
- Fat: 20g
- Carbohydrates: 8g
- Fiber: 2g
- Prep Time: 10 minutes
- Serves: 2

Recipe 5: Asian-Inspired Shrimp and Noodle Salad

Ingredients:

- 8 oz cooked shrimp, peeled and deveined
- 2 cups cooked soba noodles, cooled

- 1 cup cucumber, julienned
- 1/2 cup carrot, shredded
- 1/4 cup green onions, chopped
- 2 tablespoons soy sauce
- 1 tablespoon sesame oil
- 1 tablespoon rice vinegar
- 1 teaspoon honey
- Sesame seeds for garnish

Instructions:

1. In a large bowl, combine cooked shrimp, soba noodles, cucumber, carrot, and green onions.
2. In a small bowl, whisk together soy sauce, sesame oil, rice vinegar, and honey to make the dressing.
3. Drizzle the dressing over the salad and toss gently.
4. Garnish with sesame seeds.
5. Serve chilled.

Nutrition Information:

- Calories: 320
- Protein: 20g
- Fat: 8g
- Carbohydrates: 40g
- Fiber: 4g
- Prep Time: 15 minutes
- Cook Time: 10 minutes

- Serves: 2

Nutrient-Dense Wraps and Sandwiches

Recipe 1: Avocado Turkey Wrap

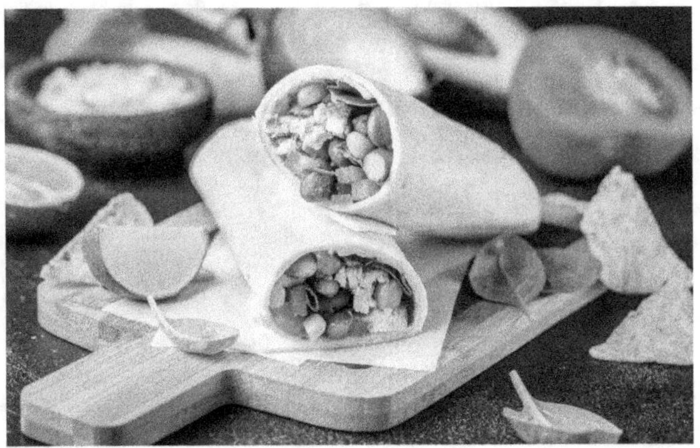

Ingredients:

- 1 whole-grain tortilla
- 3 oz sliced turkey breast
- 1/2 avocado, sliced
- 1 cup spinach leaves
- 1/4 cup cherry tomatoes, halved
- 1 tablespoon hummus
- Salt and pepper to taste

Instructions:

1. Lay the whole-grain tortilla flat.
2. Spread hummus evenly over the tortilla.

3. Layer sliced turkey, avocado, spinach, and cherry tomatoes.
4. Season with salt and pepper.
5. Roll the tortilla tightly, folding in the sides as you go.
6. Slice in half diagonally.
7. Secure with toothpicks if needed.
8. Serve immediately.

Nutrition Information:

- Calories: 380
- Protein: 20g
- Fat: 15g
- Carbohydrates: 45g
- Fiber: 10g
- Prep Time: 10 minutes
- Serves: 1

Recipe 2: Chickpea and Veggie Wrap

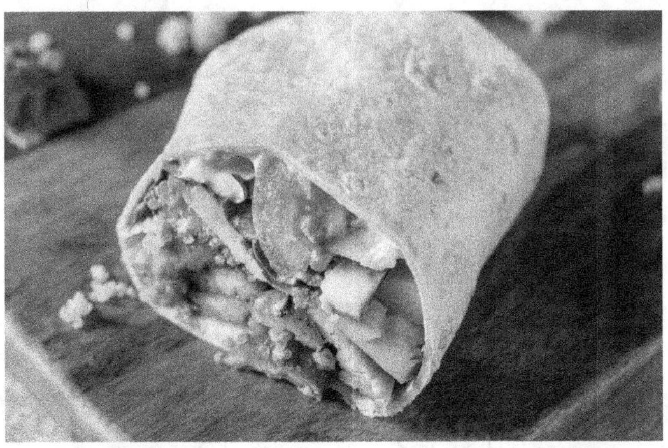

Ingredients:

- 1 whole-grain wrap
- 1/2 cup canned chickpeas, drained and rinsed
- 1/4 cup cucumber, diced
- 1/4 cup bell pepper, diced
- 2 tablespoons feta cheese, crumbled
- 1 tablespoon olive oil
- 1 tablespoon lemon juice
- 1 teaspoon dried oregano
- Salt and pepper to taste

Instructions:

1. In a bowl, combine chickpeas, cucumber, bell pepper, and feta cheese.
2. Drizzle olive oil and lemon juice over the mixture.

3. Sprinkle with dried oregano, salt, and pepper.
4. Toss to combine.
5. Lay out the whole-grain wrap.
6. Spoon the chickpea mixture onto the center of the wrap.
7. Fold in the sides and roll tightly.
8. Slice in half.
9. Serve immediately.

Nutrition Information:
- Calories: 420
- Protein: 15g
- Fat: 20g
- Carbohydrates: 50g
- Fiber: 12g
- Prep Time: 15 minutes
- Serves: 1

Recipe 3: Caprese Grilled Chicken Sandwich

Ingredients:
- 1 ciabatta roll, sliced
- 4 oz grilled chicken breast, sliced
- 1 large tomato, sliced
- 2 oz fresh mozzarella, sliced
- 1/4 cup fresh basil leaves
- 1 tablespoon balsamic glaze

- 1 tablespoon olive oil
- Salt and pepper to taste

Instructions:
1. Preheat a grill or grill pan.
2. Brush the ciabatta slices and chicken breast with olive oil.
3. Grill the chicken until cooked through, about 6-8 minutes per side.
4. Toast the ciabatta slices on the grill.
5. Assemble the sandwich by layering grilled chicken, tomato, mozzarella, and basil on the ciabatta slices.
6. Drizzle with balsamic glaze.
7. Season with salt and pepper.
8. Serve immediately.

Nutrition Information:
- Calories: 480
- Protein: 35g
- Fat: 18g
- Carbohydrates: 45g
- Fiber: 4g
- Prep Time: 20 minutes
- Cook Time: 15 minutes
- Serves: 1

Snack Ideas to Curb your Mid-Day Cravings

Snack 1: Nutty Energy Bites

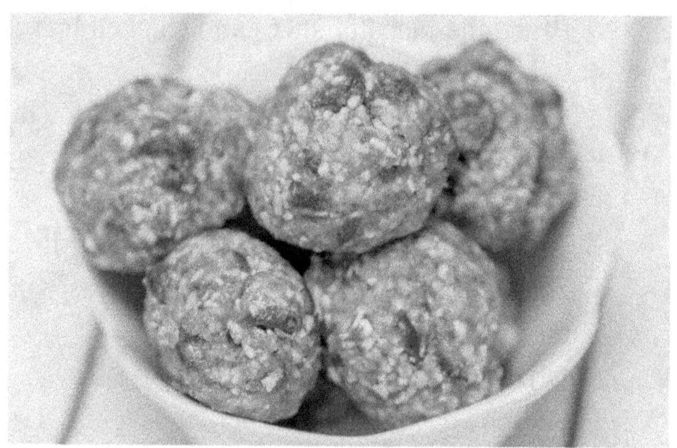

Ingredients:

- 1 cup rolled oats
- 1/2 cup nut butter (almond or peanut)
- 1/3 cup honey or maple syrup
- 1/2 cup ground flaxseed
- 1/2 cup chopped nuts (walnuts, almonds)
- 1 teaspoon vanilla extract
- Pinch of salt

Instructions:

1. In a bowl, mix rolled oats, nut butter, honey or maple syrup, ground flaxseed, chopped nuts, vanilla extract, and a pinch of salt.

2. Refrigerate the mixture for 15-30 minutes.
3. Roll the mixture into bite-sized balls.
4. Store in the refrigerator and grab a couple when hunger strikes.

Nutrition Information:

- Calories: 120 per bite
- Protein: 4g
- Fat: 8g
- Carbohydrates: 10g
- Fiber: 2g
- Prep Time: 10 minutes
- Serves: Makes 12 bites

Snack 2: Greek Yogurt Parfait

Ingredients:

- 1 cup Greek yogurt
- 1/2 cup mixed berries (strawberries, blueberries)
- 2 tablespoons granola
- Drizzle of honey

Instructions:

1. In a glass or bowl, layer Greek yogurt.
2. Add a layer of mixed berries.
3. Sprinkle granola on top.
4. Repeat the layers.
5. Finish with a drizzle of honey.

6. Enjoy this protein-packed and satisfying snack.

Nutrition Information:
- Calories: 200
- Protein: 15g
- Fat: 6g
- Carbohydrates: 25g
- Fiber: 4g
- Prep Time: 5 minutes
- Serves: 1

Snack 3: Veggie Sticks with Hummus

Ingredients:
- 1 cup baby carrots
- 1 cup cucumber sticks
- 1/2 cup cherry tomatoes
- 1/4 cup hummus

Instructions:
1. Wash and cut baby carrots, cucumber sticks, and cherry tomatoes.
2. Arrange the veggies on a plate.
3. Serve with hummus for a delicious and crunchy snack.
4. Dip and enjoy!

Nutrition Information:
- Calories: 150

- Protein: 5g
- Fat: 8g
- Carbohydrates: 18g
- Fiber: 6g
- Prep Time: 10 minutes
- Serves: 1

Snack 4: Avocado Toast with a Twist

Ingredients:
- 1 slice whole-grain bread, toasted
- 1/2 ripe avocado, mashed
- 1 teaspoon lemon juice
- Pinch of red pepper flakes
- Sprinkle of sesame seeds
- Salt and pepper to taste

Instructions:
1. Toast a slice of whole-grain bread.
2. In a bowl, mash the ripe avocado and mix it with lemon juice, red pepper flakes, salt, and pepper.
3. Spread the avocado mixture over the toasted bread.
4. Sprinkle sesame seeds on top.
5. Slice and enjoy this savory and satisfying snack.

Nutrition Information:
- Calories: 220

- Protein: 5g
- Fat: 15g
- Carbohydrates: 20g
- Fiber: 7g
- Prep Time: 5 minutes
- Serves: 1

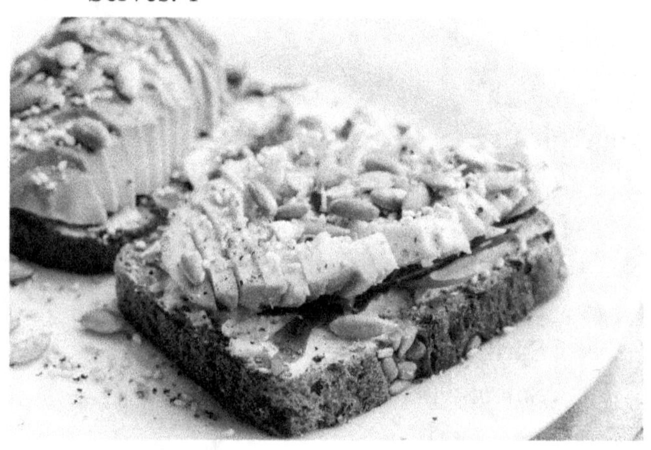

CHAPTER 5: NOURISHING DINNERS AND ENTRÉES

Balanced Plate: Lean Proteins, Veggies, and Whole Grains

Recipe 1: Grilled Chicken Quinoa Bowl

Ingredients:
- 1 cup cooked quinoa
- 6 oz grilled chicken breast, sliced
- 1 cup broccoli florets, steamed
- 1/2 cup cherry tomatoes, halved
- 1 tablespoon olive oil
- Salt and pepper to taste
- Fresh lemon wedges for garnish

Instructions:
1. Season grilled chicken with salt and pepper.
2. In a bowl, assemble cooked quinoa, grilled chicken slices, steamed broccoli, and cherry tomatoes.
3. Drizzle with olive oil.
4. Toss gently to combine.
5. Garnish with fresh lemon wedges.
6. Serve and enjoy!

Nutrition Information:

- Calories: 450
- Protein: 35g
- Fat: 15g
- Carbohydrates: 40g
- Fiber: 7g
- Prep Time: 15 minutes
- Cook Time: 15 minutes
- Serves: 2

Recipe 2: Lentil and Vegetable Stir-Fry

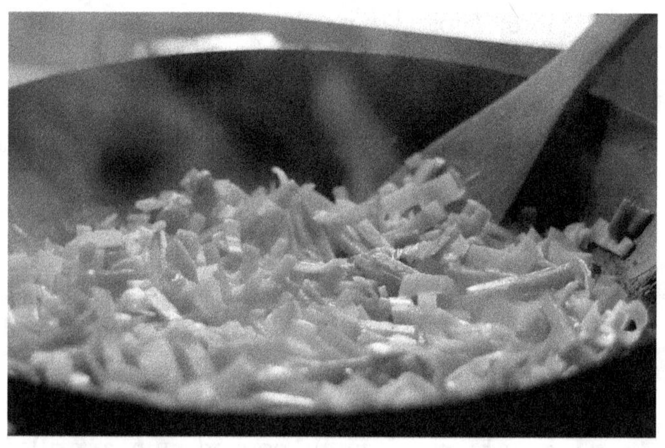

Ingredients:

- 1 cup cooked brown rice
- 1 cup cooked lentils
- 1 cup mixed bell peppers, sliced
- 1 cup snap peas
- 1 medium carrot, julienned
- 2 tablespoons soy sauce

- 1 tablespoon sesame oil
- 1 teaspoon ginger, minced
- 2 cloves garlic, minced

Instructions:

1. In a pan, sauté bell peppers, snap peas, and carrots in sesame oil until tender.
2. Add cooked lentils, cooked brown rice, soy sauce, ginger, and garlic.
3. Stir-fry for 3-5 minutes until well combined.
4. Adjust seasoning if necessary.
5. Serve hot.

Nutrition Information:

- Calories: 420
- Protein: 18g
- Fat: 8g
- Carbohydrates: 70g
- Fiber: 12g
- Prep Time: 20 minutes
- Cook Time: 15 minutes
- Serves: 2

Recipe 3: Salmon and Quinoa Stuffed Peppers

Ingredients:

- 2 large bell peppers, halved
- 8 oz salmon filet, cooked and flaked

- 1 cup cooked quinoa
- 1 cup spinach, chopped
- 1/2 cup feta cheese, crumbled
- 1 tablespoon olive oil
- Salt and pepper to taste

Instructions:
1. Preheat the oven to 375°F (190°C).
2. In a bowl, combine flaked salmon, cooked quinoa, chopped spinach, and feta cheese.
3. Drizzle with olive oil and season with salt and pepper.
4. Stuff each bell pepper half with the mixture.
5. Place stuffed peppers on a baking sheet.
6. Bake for 25-30 minutes until peppers are tender.
7. Serve warm.

Nutrition Information:
- Calories: 380
- Protein: 30g
- Fat: 16g
- Carbohydrates: 30g
- Fiber: 5g
- Prep Time: 20 minutes
- Cook Time: 30 minutes
- Serves: 2

Recipe 4: Turkey and Vegetable Quinoa Skillet

Ingredients:

- 1 cup cooked quinoa
- 8 oz ground turkey
- 1 cup zucchini, diced
- 1 cup cherry tomatoes, halved
- 1/2 cup red onion, diced
- 2 cloves garlic, minced
- 1 teaspoon olive oil
- 1 teaspoon Italian seasoning
- Salt and pepper to taste

Instructions:

1. In a skillet, heat olive oil over medium heat.
2. Add ground turkey and cook until browned.
3. Add zucchini, cherry tomatoes, red onion, and garlic.
4. Season with Italian seasoning, salt, and pepper.
5. Stir in cooked quinoa.
6. Cook for an additional 5-7 minutes until vegetables are tender.
7. Serve hot.

Nutrition Information:

- Calories: 420
- Protein: 28g

- Fat: 15g
- Carbohydrates: 45g
- Fiber: 7g
- Prep Time: 15 minutes
- Cook Time: 20 minutes
- Serves: 2

Recipe 5: Shrimp and Vegetable Brown Rice Bowl

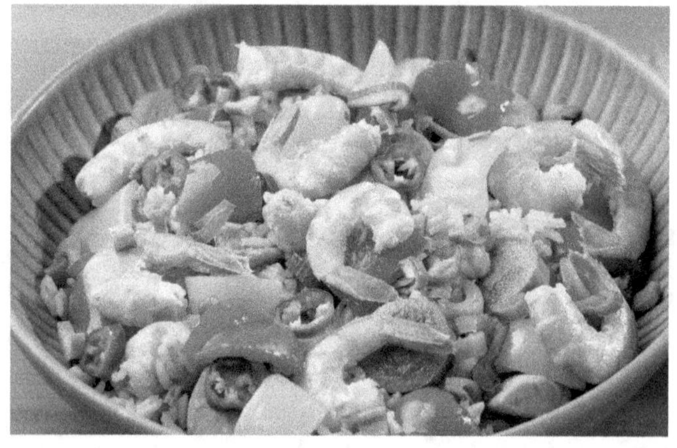

Ingredients:
- 1 cup cooked brown rice
- 8 oz shrimp, peeled and deveined
- 1 cup broccoli florets, steamed
- 1 cup bell peppers, sliced
- 1/2 cup snow peas
- 1 tablespoon soy sauce
- 1 tablespoon sesame oil

- 1 teaspoon ginger, grated
- 2 cloves garlic, minced

Instructions:

1. In a pan, sauté shrimp in sesame oil until cooked.
2. Add sliced bell peppers, steamed broccoli, and snow peas.
3. Stir in cooked brown rice.
4. Pour soy sauce over the mixture.
5. Add grated ginger and minced garlic.
6. Stir-fry for 3-5 minutes until well combined.
7. Serve hot.

Nutrition Information:

- Calories: 380
- Protein: 25g
- Fat: 8g
- Carbohydrates: 50g
- Fiber: 6g
- Prep Time: 15 minutes
- Cook Time: 10 minutes
- Serves: 2

Meatless Monday: Vegetarian and Vegan Dinner Delights

Recipe 1: Chickpea and Vegetable Stir-Fry

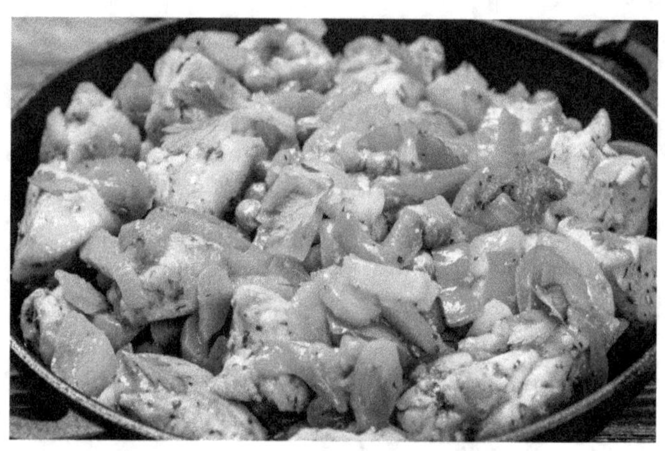

Ingredients:

- 1 can chickpeas, drained and rinsed
- 2 cups mixed vegetables (bell peppers, broccoli, snap peas)
- 2 tablespoons soy sauce
- 1 tablespoon sesame oil
- 1 tablespoon ginger, minced
- 2 cloves garlic, minced
- Brown rice for serving

Instructions:

1. In a large skillet, heat sesame oil over medium heat. Add ginger and garlic, sauté until fragrant.
2. Add mixed vegetables and chickpeas. Stir-fry until vegetables are tender yet crisp.
3. Pour soy sauce over the mixture and toss until well coated.
4. Serve over brown rice.

Nutrition Information:
- Calories: 350
- Protein: 15g
- Fat: 10g
- Carbohydrates: 50g
- Fiber: 12g
- Prep Time: 10 minutes
- Cook Time: 15 minutes
- Serves: 4

Recipe 2: Quinoa and Black Bean Stuffed Peppers

Ingredients:
- 4 bell peppers, halved and seeds removed
- 1 cup cooked quinoa
- 1 can black beans, drained and rinsed
- 1 cup corn kernels
- 1 cup diced tomatoes
- 1 teaspoon cumin

- 1 teaspoon chili powder
- Salt and pepper to taste
- Fresh cilantro for garnish

Instructions:
1. Preheat the oven to 375°F (190°C).
2. In a bowl, mix cooked quinoa, black beans, corn, diced tomatoes, cumin, chili powder, salt, and pepper.
3. Stuff each bell pepper half with the quinoa mixture.
4. Bake for 25-30 minutes or until peppers are tender.
5. Garnish with fresh cilantro before serving.

Nutrition Information:
- Calories: 280
- Protein: 12g
- Fat: 2g
- Carbohydrates: 55g
- Fiber: 12g
- Prep Time: 15 minutes
- Cook Time: 30 minutes
- Serves: 4

Recipe 3: Lentil and Vegetable Curry

Ingredients:
- 1 cup dry lentils, rinsed

- 2 cups mixed vegetables (carrots, peas, potatoes)
- 1 can coconut milk
- 1 onion, diced
- 2 cloves garlic, minced
- 1 tablespoon curry powder
- 1 teaspoon turmeric
- Salt and pepper to taste
- Fresh cilantro for garnish
- Cooked brown rice for serving

Instructions:

1. In a large pot, sauté onions and garlic until softened.
2. Add lentils, mixed vegetables, coconut milk, curry powder, turmeric, salt, and pepper.
3. Simmer until lentils and vegetables are cooked through.
4. Serve over brown rice and garnish with fresh cilantro.

Nutrition Information:

- Calories: 380
- Protein: 18g
- Fat: 15g
- Carbohydrates: 45g
- Fiber: 12g
- Prep Time: 15 minutes
- Cook Time: 40 minutes

Recipe 4: Spinach and Mushroom Vegan Pasta

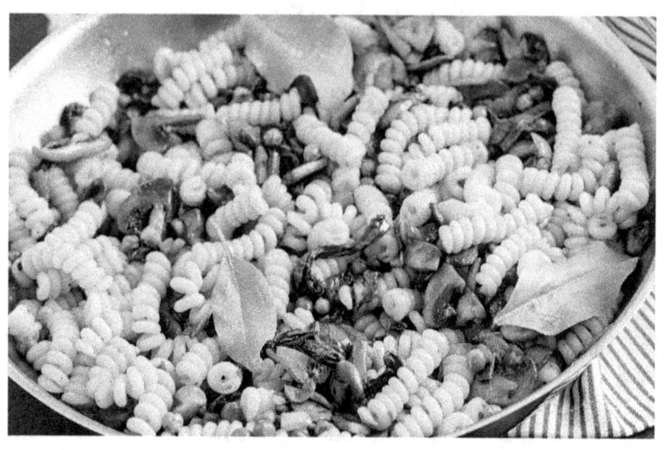

Ingredients:

- 8 oz whole wheat pasta
- 2 cups fresh spinach
- 1 cup mushrooms, sliced
- 1 can diced tomatoes
- 2 cloves garlic, minced
- 1 tablespoon olive oil
- 1 teaspoon dried oregano
- Salt and pepper to taste
- Nutritional yeast for topping

Instructions:

1. Cook pasta according to package instructions.
2. In a pan, sauté mushrooms and garlic in olive oil until mushrooms are tender.
3. Add fresh spinach and cook until wilted.
4. Stir in diced tomatoes, dried oregano, salt, and pepper.
5. Toss the cooked pasta with the vegetable mixture.
6. Top with nutritional yeast before serving.

Nutrition Information:
- Calories: 320
- Protein: 12g
- Fat: 8g
- Carbohydrates: 55g
- Fiber: 10g
- Prep Time: 10 minutes
- Cook Time: 20 minutes
- Serves: 4

Recipe 5: Sweet Potato and Chickpea Curry

Ingredients:
- 2 large sweet potatoes, peeled and diced
- 1 can chickpeas, drained and rinsed
- 1 can coconut milk
- 1 onion, finely chopped

- 2 tablespoons red curry paste
- 1 teaspoon ground coriander
- 1 teaspoon cumin
- Salt and pepper to taste
- Fresh cilantro for garnish
- Cooked quinoa for serving

Instructions:
1. In a large pot, sauté onions until translucent.
2. Add sweet potatoes, chickpeas, coconut milk, red curry paste, ground coriander, cumin, salt, and pepper.
3. Simmer until sweet potatoes are tender.
4. Serve over cooked quinoa and garnish with fresh cilantro.

Nutrition Information:
- Calories: 400
- Protein: 14g
- Fat: 20g
- Carbohydrates: 50g
- Fiber: 10g
- Prep Time: 20 minutes
- Cook Time: 30 minutes
- Serves: 4

Easy One-Pot Meals for Busy Weeknights

Recipe 1: One-Pot Chicken and Vegetable Stir-Fry

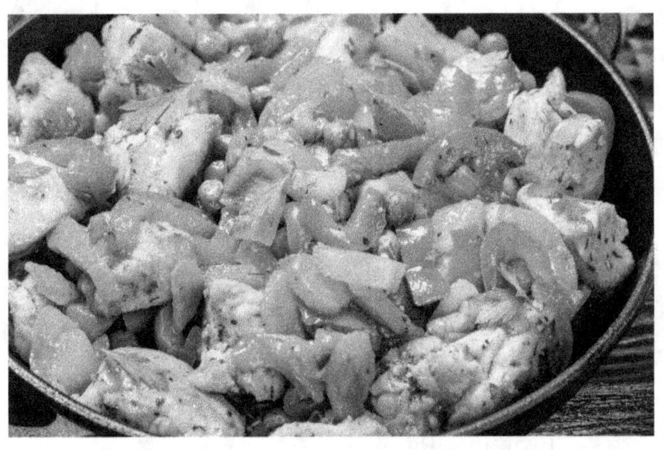

Ingredients:

- 1 lb boneless, skinless chicken breasts, thinly sliced
- 2 cups broccoli florets
- 1 bell pepper, thinly sliced
- 1 carrot, julienned
- 3 tablespoons soy sauce
- 2 tablespoons oyster sauce
- 1 tablespoon sesame oil
- 2 cloves garlic, minced
- 1 tablespoon ginger, grated

- 2 cups cooked brown rice

Instructions:
1. In a large skillet, heat sesame oil over medium-high heat.
2. Add chicken and cook until browned.
3. Add broccoli, bell pepper, and carrot. Stir in garlic and ginger.
4. Pour soy sauce and oyster sauce over the mixture, stirring well.
5. Cover and simmer until vegetables are tender.
6. Serve over cooked brown rice.

Nutrition Information:
- Calories: 400
- Protein: 30g
- Fat: 12g
- Carbohydrates: 45g
- Fiber: 8g
- Prep Time: 10 minutes
- Cook Time: 20 minutes
- Serves: 4

Recipe 2: One-Pot Tomato Basil Pasta

Ingredients:
- 8 oz linguine
- 2 cups cherry tomatoes, halved
- 3 cloves garlic, thinly sliced

- 1/4 teaspoon red pepper flakes
- 2 tablespoons olive oil
- 4 cups vegetable broth
- Salt and pepper to taste
- Fresh basil leaves for garnish
- Grated Parmesan cheese (optional)

Instructions:

1. In a large pot, combine linguine, cherry tomatoes, garlic, red pepper flakes, olive oil, and vegetable broth.
2. Season with salt and pepper.
3. Bring to a boil, then reduce heat and simmer until pasta is cooked and broth is absorbed.
4. Garnish with fresh basil and Parmesan cheese if desired.

Nutrition Information:

- Calories: 350
- Protein: 9g
- Fat: 8g
- Carbohydrates: 60g
- Fiber: 4g
- Prep Time: 5 minutes
- Cook Time: 15 minutes
- Serves: 3

Recipe 3: One-Pot Chickpea and Spinach Curry

Ingredients:
- 1 can chickpeas, drained and rinsed
- 1 onion, finely chopped
- 2 tomatoes, diced
- 2 cups spinach leaves
- 1 can coconut milk
- 2 tablespoons curry powder
- 1 teaspoon cumin
- 1 teaspoon turmeric
- Salt and pepper to taste
- Cooked quinoa or rice for serving

Instructions:
1. In a large pot, sauté onions until translucent.
2. Add tomatoes, chickpeas, spinach, coconut milk, curry powder, cumin, and turmeric.
3. Season with salt and pepper.
4. Simmer until spinach wilts and flavors meld.
5. Serve over cooked quinoa or rice.

Nutrition Information:
- Calories: 420
- Protein: 15g
- Fat: 20g
- Carbohydrates: 50g
- Fiber: 14g

- Prep Time: 15 minutes
- Cook Time: 25 minutes
- Serves: 4

Recipe 4: One-Pot Lemon Garlic Shrimp and Quinoa

Ingredients:
- 1 lb shrimp, peeled and deveined
- 1 cup quinoa, rinsed
- 2 cups chicken broth
- 1 lemon, juiced and zested
- 3 cloves garlic, minced
- 1 teaspoon dried thyme
- 1 cup cherry tomatoes, halved
- Fresh parsley for garnish

Instructions:
1. In a large pot, combine quinoa, chicken broth, lemon juice, lemon zest, garlic, and thyme.
2. Bring to a boil, then reduce heat, cover, and simmer until quinoa is cooked.
3. Add shrimp and cherry tomatoes, cooking until shrimp are pink.
4. Garnish with fresh parsley before serving.

Nutrition Information:
- Calories: 380

- Protein: 35g
- Fat: 6g
- Carbohydrates: 45g
- Fiber: 6g
- Prep Time: 10 minutes
- Cook Time: 20 minutes
- Serves: 3

Recipe 5: One-Pot Lentil and Vegetable Stew

Ingredients:
- 1 cup dried green lentils, rinsed
- 1 onion, chopped
- 2 carrots, diced
- 2 celery stalks, sliced
- 3 cloves garlic, minced
- 1 can diced tomatoes
- 4 cups vegetable broth
- 1 teaspoon cumin
- 1 teaspoon smoked paprika
- Salt and pepper to taste
- Fresh cilantro for garnish

Instructions:
1. In a large pot, sauté onions, carrots, celery, and garlic until softened.
2. Add lentils, diced tomatoes, vegetable broth, cumin, and smoked paprika.

3. Season with salt and pepper.
4. Simmer until lentils are tender.
5. Garnish with fresh cilantro before serving.

Nutrition Information:
- Calories: 320
- Protein: 18g
- Fat: 2g
- Carbohydrates: 60g
- Fiber: 16g
- Prep Time: 15 minutes
- Cook Time: 30 minutes
- Serves: 4

Recipe 6: One-Pot Chicken and Quinoa Chili

Ingredients:
- 1 lb ground chicken
- 1 onion, diced
- 2 bell peppers, chopped
- 3 cloves garlic, minced
- 1 can black beans, drained and rinsed
- 1 can diced tomatoes
- 1 cup frozen corn
- 2 tablespoons chili powder
- 1 teaspoon cumin
- Salt and pepper to taste
- Avocado and shredded cheese for topping

Instructions:

1. In a large pot, cook ground chicken until browned.
2. Add onions, bell peppers, and garlic, sautéing until softened.
3. Stir in black beans, diced tomatoes, frozen corn, chili powder, and cumin.
4. Season with salt and pepper.
5. Simmer until flavors meld.
6. Serve topped with avocado and shredded cheese.

Nutrition Information:

- Calories: 380
- Protein: 30g
- Fat: 12g
- Carbohydrates: 40g
- Fiber: 10g
- Prep Time: 10 minutes
- Cook Time: 25 minutes
- Serves: 4

CHAPTER 6: HEALTHY DESSERTS AND INDULGENT TREATS

Guilt-Free Desserts to Satisfy Your Sweet Tooth

Recipe 1: Chocolate Avocado Mousse

Ingredients:
- 2 ripe avocados
- 1/4 cup cocoa powder
- 1/4 cup maple syrup or honey
- 1 teaspoon vanilla extract
- Pinch of salt
- Fresh berries for garnish

Instructions:
1. Scoop out the avocados and place them in a blender.
2. Add cocoa powder, maple syrup, vanilla extract, and a pinch of salt.
3. Blend until smooth and creamy.
4. Refrigerate for at least 1 hour before serving.
5. Garnish with fresh berries before serving.

Nutrition Information:

- Calories: 180
- Protein: 3g
- Fat: 14g
- Carbohydrates: 18g
- Fiber: 6g
- Prep Time: 10 minutes
- Serves: 4

Recipe 2: Greek Yogurt and Berry Popsicles

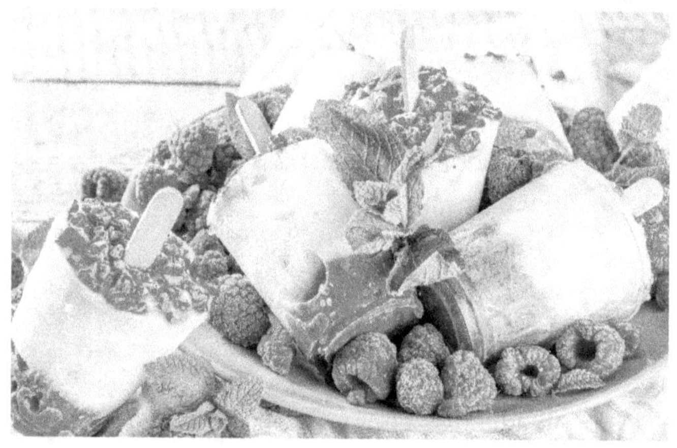

Ingredients:

- 1 cup Greek yogurt
- 1 cup mixed berries (strawberries, blueberries, raspberries)
- 2 tablespoons honey
- 1 teaspoon vanilla extract

Instructions:

1. In a bowl, mix Greek yogurt, honey, and vanilla extract.
2. Layer the yogurt mixture and mixed berries in popsicle molds.
3. Insert popsicle sticks and freeze for at least 4 hours.
4. Enjoy these refreshing guilt-free popsicles.

Nutrition Information:

- Calories: 70
- Protein: 5g
- Fat: 2g
- Carbohydrates: 12g
- Fiber: 2g
- Prep Time: 15 minutes
- Freeze Time: 4 hours
- Serves: 6

Recipe 3: Baked Cinnamon Apple Chips

Ingredients:

- 2 apples, thinly sliced
- 1 tablespoon cinnamon
- 1 tablespoon coconut sugar (optional)

Instructions:

1. Preheat the oven to 225°F (110°C).
2. Arrange the apple slices on a parchment-lined baking sheet.

3. Sprinkle it with cinnamon and coconut sugar.
4. Bake for 2-3 hours until the chips are crisp.
5. Allow them to cool before serving.

Nutrition Information:
- Calories: 50
- Protein: 0.5g
- Fat: 0.2g
- Carbohydrates: 13g
- Fiber: 2.5g
- Prep Time: 15 minutes
- Bake Time: 2-3 hours
- Serves: 4

Recipe 4: No-Bake Energy Bites

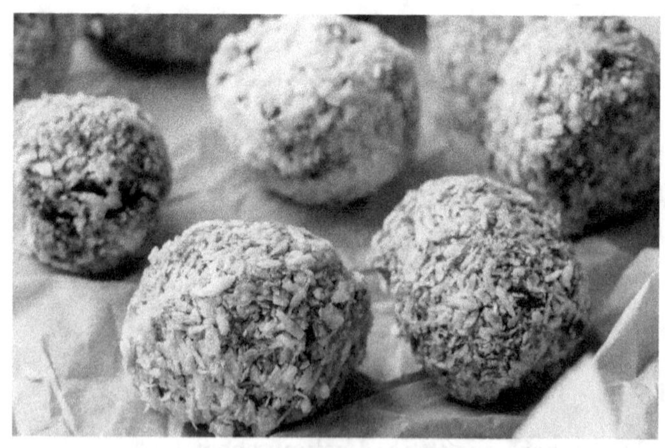

Ingredients:

- 1 cup rolled oats
- 1/2 cup almond butter
- 1/3 cup honey
- 1/2 cup ground flaxseed
- 1/2 cup dark chocolate chips
- 1 teaspoon vanilla extract

Instructions:

1. In a bowl, mix rolled oats, almond butter, honey, ground flaxseed, chocolate chips, and vanilla extract.
2. Refrigerate for 30 minutes.
3. Roll the mixture into bite-sized balls.
4. Refrigerate for an additional 30 minutes before serving.

Nutrition Information:

- Calories: 120
- Protein: 3g
- Fat: 7g
- Carbohydrates: 12g
- Fiber: 2.5g
- Prep Time: 15 minutes
- Chill Time: 1 hour
- Serves: 12

Recipe 5: Coconut Chia Seed Pudding

Ingredients:
- 1/4 cup chia seeds
- 1 cup coconut milk
- 1 tablespoon maple syrup or honey
- 1/2 teaspoon vanilla extract
- Fresh fruit for topping

Instructions:
1. In a bowl, mix chia seeds, coconut milk, maple syrup, and vanilla extract.
2. Refrigerate for at least 4 hours or overnight.
3. Stir well before serving.
4. Top with fresh fruit before serving.

Nutrition Information:
- Calories: 180
- Protein: 3g
- Fat: 12g
- Carbohydrates: 18g
- Fiber: 6g
- Prep Time: 5 minutes
- Chill Time: 4 hours
- Serves: 2

Fruit-Based Desserts and Homemade Frozen Treats

Ingredients:
- 2 cups ripe mango chunks
- 1 cup coconut milk
- 2 tablespoons honey or maple syrup
- 1 teaspoon vanilla extract

Instructions:
1. Blend mango chunks, coconut milk, honey (or maple syrup), and vanilla extract until smooth.
2. Pour the mixture into popsicle molds.
3. Insert popsicle sticks and freeze for at least 4 hours or until solid.
4. Run the molds under warm water to release the popsicles.
5. Enjoy these tropical delights!

Nutrition Information:
- Calories: 120
- Protein: 1g
- Fat: 5g
- Carbohydrates: 20g
- Prep Time: 10 minutes
- Freeze Time: 4 hours

- Serves: 6

Recipe 2: Berry Medley Parfait

Ingredients:
- 1 cup mixed berries (strawberries, blueberries, raspberries)
- 1 cup vanilla Greek yogurt
- 1/2 cup granola
- Drizzle of honey

Instructions:
1. In a glass or bowl, layer mixed berries.
2. Spoon vanilla Greek yogurt over the berries.
3. Sprinkle granola on top.
4. Repeat the layers.
5. Finish with a drizzle of honey.
6. Refrigerate for 30 minutes before serving.

Nutrition Information:
- Calories: 250
- Protein: 10g
- Fat: 6g
- Carbohydrates: 40g
- Fiber: 5g
- Prep Time: 10 minutes
- Serves: 2

Recipe 3: Watermelon Mint Sorbet

Ingredients:
- 4 cups seedless watermelon, diced
- 1/4 cup fresh mint leaves
- 2 tablespoons lime juice
- 2 tablespoons honey or agave syrup

Instructions:
1. Blend watermelon, mint leaves, lime juice, and honey (or agave syrup) until smooth.
2. Pour the mixture into a shallow dish.
3. Freeze for 2-3 hours, stirring every 30 minutes with a fork to break up ice crystals.
4. Once fully frozen, scoop into bowls and serve.

Nutrition Information:
- Calories: 90
- Protein: 1g
- Fat: 0g
- Carbohydrates: 24g
- Prep Time: 15 minutes
- Freeze Time: 3 hours
- Serves: 4

Recipe 4: Pineapple Coconut Ice Cream

Ingredients:
- 2 cups frozen pineapple chunks

- 1 can (13.5 oz) coconut milk, chilled
- 1/4 cup shredded coconut (optional)
- 2 tablespoons maple syrup

Instructions:

1. In a blender, combine frozen pineapple chunks, chilled coconut milk, shredded coconut (if using), and maple syrup.
2. Blend until smooth and creamy.
3. Transfer to a freezer-safe container and freeze for 2-3 hours.
4. Scoop and serve, garnishing with additional shredded coconut if desired.

Nutrition Information:

- Calories: 220
- Protein: 2g
- Fat: 15g
- Carbohydrates: 22g
- Fiber: 2g
- Prep Time: 10 minutes
- Freeze Time: 3 hours
- Serves: 4

CHAPTER 7: WORKOUT FUEL AND RECOVERY

Pre- and Post-Workout Snacks and Meals

Recipe 1: Pre-Workout Energy Bites

Ingredients:
- 1 cup rolled oats
- 1/2 cup almond butter
- 1/4 cup honey
- 1/4 cup ground flaxseeds
- 1/2 cup chocolate chips
- 1 teaspoon vanilla extract
- Pinch of salt

Instructions:
1. In a bowl, mix rolled oats, almond butter, honey, ground flaxseeds, chocolate chips, vanilla extract, and a pinch of salt.
2. Form small, bite-sized balls from the mixture.
3. Place the energy bites in the refrigerator for at least 30 minutes.
4. Enjoy a couple of bites about 30 minutes before your workout.

Nutrition Information:

- Calories: 120 per bite
- Protein: 4g
- Fat: 7g
- Carbohydrates: 12g
- Fiber: 2g
- Prep Time: 10 minutes
- Serves: 12 bites

Recipe 2: Grilled Chicken and Quinoa Salad (Post-Workout)

Ingredients:

- 1 cup cooked quinoa
- 6 oz grilled chicken breast, sliced
- 1 cup cherry tomatoes, halved
- 1/2 cucumber, diced
- 1/4 cup feta cheese, crumbled
- 2 tablespoons olive oil
- 1 tablespoon balsamic vinegar
- Salt and pepper to taste

Instructions:

1. In a bowl, combine quinoa, grilled chicken, cherry tomatoes, cucumber, and feta cheese.
2. In a small bowl, whisk together olive oil, balsamic vinegar, salt, and pepper.
3. Drizzle the dressing over the salad and toss gently.

4. Serve as a satisfying post-workout meal.

Nutrition Information:
- Calories: 450
- Protein: 35g
- Fat: 20g
- Carbohydrates: 30g
- Fiber: 5g
- Prep Time: 15 minutes
- Cook Time: 15 minutes
- Serves: 2

Recipe 3: Banana and Almond Butter Toast (Pre-Workout)

Ingredients:
- 2 slices whole-grain bread
- 2 tablespoons almond butter
- 1 banana, sliced
- Drizzle of honey
- Pinch of cinnamon

Instructions:
1. Toast the whole-grain bread slices.
2. Spread almond butter evenly on each slice.
3. Arrange banana slices on top.
4. Drizzle with honey and sprinkle with a pinch of cinnamon.

5. Enjoy this quick and energizing pre-workout snack.

Nutrition Information:
- Calories: 300
- Protein: 8g
- Fat: 12g
- Carbohydrates: 40g
- Fiber: 6g
- Prep Time: 5 minutes
- Serves: 2

Recipe 4: Greek Yogurt Parfait (Post-Workout)

Ingredients:
- 1 cup Greek yogurt
- 1/2 cup mixed berries (strawberries, blueberries, raspberries)
- 1/4 cup granola
- 1 tablespoon honey
- Chopped nuts for garnish

Instructions:
1. In a glass or bowl, layer Greek yogurt, mixed berries, and granola.
2. Drizzle with honey.
3. Garnish with chopped nuts.

4. A delicious and protein-packed post-workout treat.

Nutrition Information:
- Calories: 280
- Protein: 18g
- Fat: 8g
- Carbohydrates: 35g
- Fiber: 4g
- Prep Time: 5 minutes
- Serves: 1

Recipe 5: Turkey and Avocado Wrap (Pre-Workout)

Ingredients:
- 1 whole-grain wrap
- 4 oz turkey breast slices
- 1/2 avocado, sliced
- Handful of spinach leaves
- 1 tablespoon hummus

Instructions:
1. Lay the whole-grain wrap on a flat surface.
2. Spread hummus evenly on the wrap.
3. Layer turkey slices, avocado slices, and spinach leaves.
4. Roll the wrap tightly and cut it in half.

5. A protein-rich pre-workout snack that's easy to prepare.

Nutrition Information:
- Calories: 350
- Protein: 25g
- Fat: 15g
- Carbohydrates: 30g
- Fiber: 8g
- Prep Time: 10 minutes
- Serves: 1

Recipe 6: Berry Protein Smoothie (Post-Workout)

Ingredients:
- 1 cup mixed berries (strawberries, blueberries, raspberries)
- 1 scoop vanilla protein powder
- 1 cup almond milk
- 1 tablespoon almond butter
- Ice cubes

Instructions:
1. In a blender, combine mixed berries, vanilla protein powder, almond milk, and almond butter.
2. Blend until smooth.

3. Add ice cubes and blend again for a refreshing post-workout smoothie.

Nutrition Information:
- Calories: 280
- Protein: 25g
- Fat: 12g
- Carbohydrates: 20g
- Fiber: 5g
- Prep Time: 5 minutes
- Serves: 1

Hydration and the Role of Water in Weight Loss

Drink Water Before Meals: Consuming a glass of water before meals can help control appetite and prevent overeating. It also ensures you stay hydrated while enjoying your meals.

Recipe 1: Citrus Infused Detox Water

Ingredients:
- 1 lemon, sliced
- 1 lime, sliced
- 1 orange, sliced
- 8-10 fresh mint leaves
- 1 liter of cold water
- Ice cubes (optional)

Instructions:

1. In a pitcher, combine lemon slices, lime slices, orange slices, and fresh mint leaves.
2. Fill the pitcher with cold water.
3. Allow the water to infuse in the refrigerator for at least 2 hours, or overnight for stronger flavor.
4. Serve over ice cubes if desired.
5. Enjoy this refreshing citrus-infused water throughout the day to stay hydrated.

Nutrition Information:

- Calories: 10
- Prep Time: 5 minutes
- Serves: 4

Recipe 2: Cucumber Mint Spa Water

Ingredients:

- 1 cucumber, thinly sliced
- 1/2 cup fresh mint leaves
- 1 tablespoon fresh lime juice
- 1 liter of cold water
- Ice cubes (optional)

Instructions:

1. In a pitcher, combine cucumber slices, fresh mint leaves, and lime juice.
2. Fill the pitcher with cold water.

3. Allow the water to infuse in the refrigerator for at least 1 hour.
4. Serve over ice cubes if desired.
5. Experience the revitalizing taste of this cucumber mint spa water for a hydrating treat.

Nutrition Information:
- Calories: 5
- Prep Time: 5 minutes
- Serves: 4

Recipe 3: Watermelon Basil Cooler

Ingredients:
- 2 cups fresh watermelon, cubed
- 1/4 cup fresh basil leaves
- 1 tablespoon fresh lemon juice
- 1 liter of cold water
- Ice cubes (optional)

Instructions:
1. In a blender, combine fresh watermelon cubes, basil leaves, and lemon juice.
2. Blend until smooth.
3. Strain the mixture to remove pulp.
4. In a pitcher, mix the watermelon and basil juice with cold water.
5. Refrigerate for at least 1 hour to enhance the flavors.

6. Serve over ice cubes if desired.
7. Indulge in the sweet and herbaceous notes of this watermelon basil cooler.

Nutrition Information:
- Calories: 40
- Prep Time: 15 minutes
- Serves: 4

Recipe 4: Green Tea and Peach Infusion

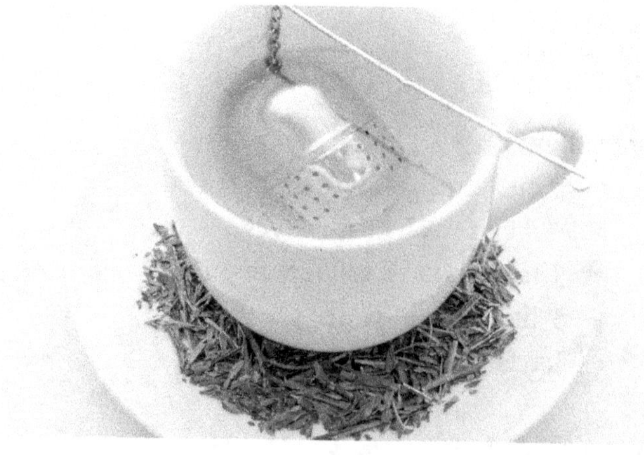

Ingredients:

- 2 green tea bags
- 2 peaches, sliced
- 1 tablespoon honey (optional)
- 1.5 liters of hot water (not boiling)
- Ice cubes

Instructions:

1. Steep green tea bags in hot water for 3-5 minutes.
2. Remove tea bags and let the tea cool to room temperature.
3. In a pitcher, combine sliced peaches, cooled green tea, and honey.
4. Refrigerate for at least 2 hours.
5. Serve over ice cubes.

Nutrition Information:

- Calories: 15
- Prep Time: 10 minutes
- Serves: 4

Recipe 5: Berry Blast Hydration Smoothie

Ingredients:

- 1 cup mixed berries (strawberries, blueberries, raspberries)
- 1 cup coconut water
- 1/2 cup plain Greek yogurt
- 1 tablespoon chia seeds
- Ice cubes

Instructions:

1. Blend mixed berries, coconut water, Greek yogurt, and chia seeds until smooth.
2. Add ice cubes and blend again.
3. Pour into glasses and enjoy this hydrating berry smoothie.

Nutrition Information:

- Calories: 120
- Prep Time: 7 minutes
- Serves: 2

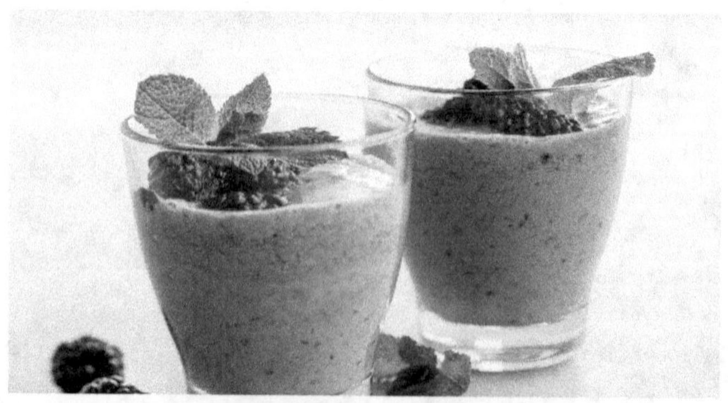

CHAPTER 8: LIFESTYLE AND MINDSET SHIFTS

The Power of Routine: Building Healthy Habits

The power of routine lies in its ability to shape our daily lives, molding behaviors into habits that can profoundly impact our well-being. Building healthy habits through consistent routines is a transformative journey. By establishing a structured framework, individuals can seamlessly integrate positive behaviors such as regular exercise, balanced nutrition, and sufficient sleep into their lives. The repetitive nature of routines not only fosters discipline but also reduces decision fatigue, making it easier to prioritize health. Whether it's morning workouts, mindful meal preparation, or a calming bedtime ritual, these routines become the foundation for a healthier lifestyle. Harnessing the power of routine empowers individuals to achieve long-term goals, cultivating a sustainable and holistic approach to well-being.

Stress Management and Mindful Eating Practices

In the fast-paced world we navigate, stress management and mindful eating practices are integral components of maintaining overall well-being. Stress often triggers unhealthy eating habits, leading to overconsumption and poor food choices. Incorporating mindfulness into eating habits offers a powerful tool for stress management. Mindful eating involves being fully present during meals, paying attention to sensory experiences, and savoring each bite. By cultivating awareness of hunger and fullness cues, individuals can make conscious food choices, preventing stress-induced emotional eating. Taking a moment to appreciate the colors, textures, and flavors of each meal promotes a healthier relationship with food.

In parallel, stress management techniques complement mindful eating. Practices such as deep breathing, meditation, and regular exercise help reduce stress levels, preventing the cascade of negative impacts on dietary choices. Building a repertoire of stress-relief strategies empowers individuals to respond to life's challenges with resilience and make mindful decisions about their well-being.

The synergy between stress management and mindful eating creates a harmonious approach to health. By fostering awareness in both areas, individuals can navigate stressors with a sense of control, making choices that contribute to not only physical health but also mental and emotional balance.

Staying Motivated on Your Weight Loss Journey

Embarking on a weight loss journey requires not just dedication, but a consistent wellspring of motivation. Here are key strategies to help you stay inspired and committed throughout your transformative path:

1. Set Realistic Goals: Establish achievable, measurable, and time-bound goals. Break them into smaller milestones, celebrating each achievement along the way. Realistic goals foster a sense of accomplishment and keep motivation high.

2. Visualize Success: Create a mental image of your future self and the benefits of achieving your weight loss goals. Visualizing success can serve as a powerful motivator, helping you stay focused on the positive outcomes.

3. Track Your Progress: Keep a record of your journey, whether through a journal, photos, or a mobile app. Tracking your progress not only provides tangible evidence of success but also serves as a reminder of how far you've come.

4. Diversify Your Routine: Prevent monotony by incorporating variety into your fitness and nutrition routines. Trying new exercises or experimenting with different healthy recipes can keep things interesting and stoke motivation.

5. Seek Support: Share your goals with friends, family, or join a community with similar objectives. Encouragement, shared experiences, and accountability from a support system can be invaluable during challenging moments.

6. Celebrate Non-Scale Victories: Recognize achievements beyond the scale. Improved energy levels, better sleep, or increased stamina are victories worth celebrating and can sustain motivation even if weight loss plateaus.

7. Reward Yourself: Establish a system of rewards for achieving milestones. These rewards don't have to be food-related; they could include a spa day, a new workout outfit, or a weekend getaway.

8. Educate Yourself: Stay informed about nutrition, fitness, and wellness. Knowledge empowers you to make informed decisions, understand your body, and appreciate the science behind your weight loss journey.

9. Practice Self-Compassion: Understand that setbacks are a natural part of the process. Be kind to yourself, learn from challenges, and use them as opportunities for growth rather than reasons to give up.

10. Visual and Written Affirmations: Create visual or written affirmations that resonate with your goals. Place them where you can see them daily to reinforce positive thoughts and intentions.

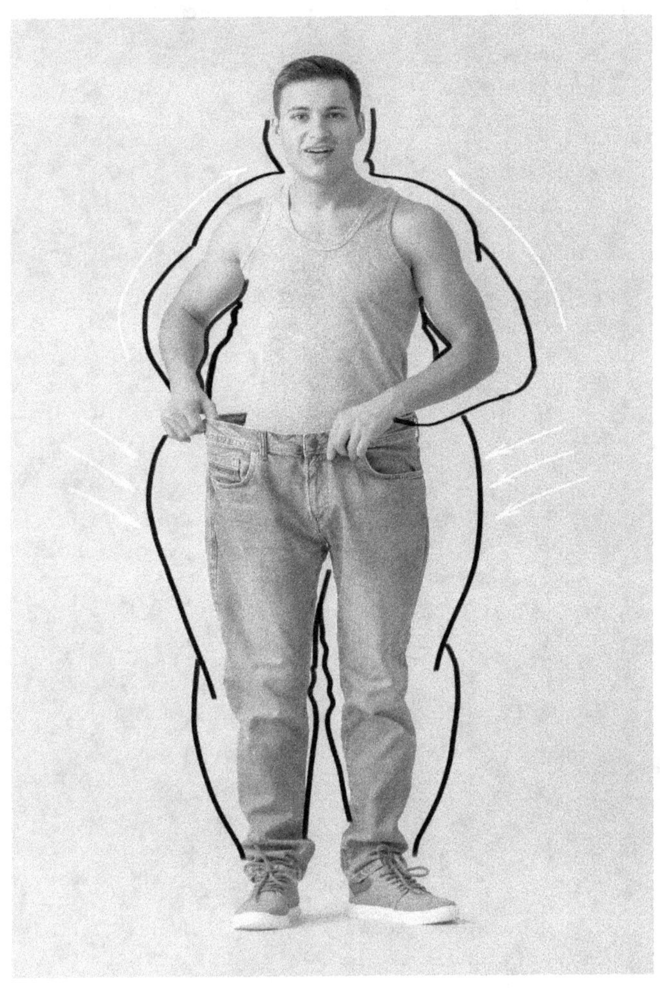

WEIGHT LOSS TIPS

Drink more water

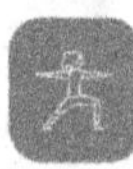
Exercise daily

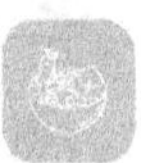
Eat healthy food

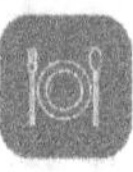
Eat when hungry

CHAPTER 9: LONG-TERM SUCCESS AND MAINTENANCE

Tips for Sustaining Weight Loss Results

Achieving weight loss is a commendable accomplishment, but maintaining those results over the long term requires ongoing dedication and a sustainable approach. Here are essential tips for sustaining weight loss success:

1. **Establish Realistic Habits:**
   - Gradually incorporate sustainable habits into your routine. Establishing realistic dietary and exercise practices ensures they become a permanent part of your lifestyle.

2. **Embrace Balance:**
   - Avoid extreme diets or restrictive eating patterns. Embrace a balanced approach that includes a variety of nutrient-dense foods, allowing for occasional treats without guilt.

3. **Regular Physical Activity:**
   - Maintain a consistent exercise routine. Choose activities you enjoy to make fitness an integral part of your life. Regular

physical activity supports weight maintenance and overall well-being.

4. Mindful Eating:

- Continue practicing mindful eating. Be aware of hunger and fullness cues, savor each bite, and remain attuned to your body's needs. This approach fosters a healthier relationship with food.

5. Stay Hydrated:

- Water is essential for overall health and can aid in weight maintenance. Stay hydrated throughout the day to support bodily functions and prevent dehydration, which can sometimes be mistaken for hunger.

6. Monitor Portion Sizes:

- Be mindful of portion sizes, especially when dining out. Pay attention to hunger cues and avoid overeating. Using smaller plates can help control portions.

7. Regular Check-Ins:

- Periodically reassess your goals and progress. Regular check-ins help you stay accountable and make necessary adjustments to your plan as circumstances change.

8. Build a Support System:

- Maintain a strong support system. Friends, family, or accountability partners can provide encouragement, share experiences, and offer valuable insights to help you stay on track.

9. **Incorporate Fun Activities:**
  - Make health and wellness enjoyable. Engage in activities you love, whether it's dancing, hiking, or trying new fitness classes. Enjoying the journey makes it more likely to be sustainable.

10. **Plan Ahead:**
  - Plan meals and snacks in advance to avoid impulsive food choices. Having healthy options readily available reduces the likelihood of resorting to convenience foods.

11. **Manage Stress:**
  - Implement stress-management techniques such as meditation, deep breathing, or yoga. Chronic stress can impact weight, so fostering stress resilience is crucial for long-term success.

12. **Celebrate Successes:**
  - Acknowledge and celebrate your achievements. Recognizing your efforts, no matter how small, reinforces positive behaviors and helps maintain motivation.

13. **Continuous Learning:**
  - Stay informed about nutrition, fitness, and overall health. Continuously educate yourself to make informed choices and adapt your lifestyle to evolving needs.

Integrating Exercise and Physical Activity into Your Lifestyle

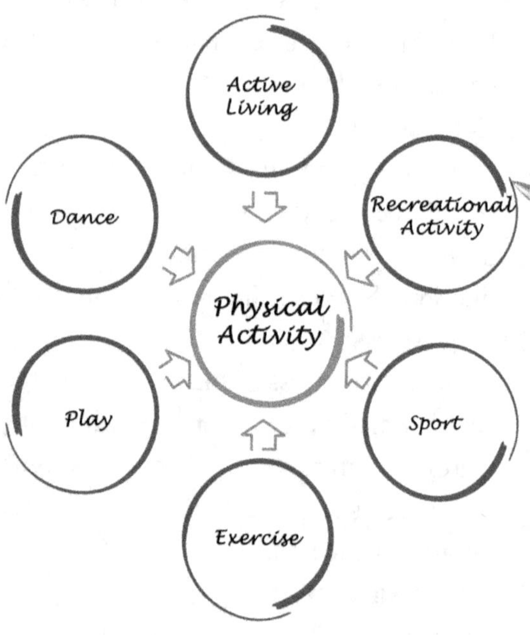

Integrating exercise and physical activity into your lifestyle is a cornerstone of overall health and well-being. Rather than viewing it as a separate task, consider it an integral part of your daily routine, seamlessly woven into the fabric of your life.

Start by identifying activities you genuinely enjoy, whether it's walking, cycling, dancing, or playing a sport. Finding joy in your chosen activities makes them more sustainable and increases the likelihood of incorporating them into your routine. Aim for at least 150 minutes of moderate-intensity aerobic exercise per week, complemented by strength training exercises at least twice a week.

Incorporate physical activity into your daily life by choosing stairs over elevators, walking or biking instead of driving short distances, or taking short breaks to stretch and move throughout the day. Establish a consistent schedule that aligns with your natural rhythm, making it easier to form a habit.

The benefits of regular exercise extend beyond weight management, encompassing improved mood, enhanced cardiovascular health, and increased energy levels. By integrating exercise into your lifestyle, you not only prioritize your physical health but also cultivate a positive mindset and an enduring commitment to your overall well-being.

Celebrating Milestones and Setting New Goals

Celebrating milestones and setting new goals is a vital aspect of personal growth and motivation. Whether in the realm of weight loss, career achievements, or personal development, acknowledging and commemorating milestones fuels a sense of accomplishment. Take the time to reflect on the journey, recognizing the effort and dedication invested in reaching each milestone. Celebrations need not be extravagant; they can be as simple as treating yourself to a favorite activity or expressing gratitude for the progress made. Concurrently, setting new goals invigorates the spirit, providing a roadmap for continued growth. Establish realistic, challenging objectives that align with your aspirations, fostering a continuous cycle of self-improvement. This combination of celebration and goal-setting creates a dynamic, forward-moving trajectory, ensuring a fulfilling and purposeful journey through life's endeavors.

CONCLUSION

Embracing Your New Relationship with Food

Embracing your new relationship with food is a transformative and empowering journey. Shift the focus from restrictive diets to a positive, mindful approach centered around nourishment and enjoyment. Cultivate an awareness of hunger and fullness, savoring the diverse flavors and textures of nutritious meals. View food as a source of energy and vitality, supporting your overall well-being. Allow flexibility in your choices, understanding that occasional indulgences are part of a balanced lifestyle. Release guilt associated with eating and foster self-compassion. By embracing a holistic and positive connection with food, you embark on a sustainable path that not only promotes physical health but also nourishes your mental and emotional resilience, fostering a harmonious and joyful relationship with the nourishment your body deserves.

Looking Ahead: Your Continued Journey to Wellness

Looking ahead, your continued journey to wellness is an ongoing adventure of self-discovery and personal growth. Reflect on the strides you've made in your pursuit of a healthier lifestyle, celebrating both small victories and significant milestones. As you navigate this path, acknowledge that wellness is a dynamic and evolving concept, encompassing physical, mental, and emotional dimensions.

Set new goals that resonate with your aspirations, promoting balance and sustainability. Whether refining fitness routines, exploring new forms of self-care, or fostering mindful eating habits, each step contributes to a holistic sense of well-being. Embrace the notion that wellness is a lifelong commitment, marked by continuous learning and adaptation.

Cultivate resilience in the face of challenges, recognizing that setbacks are natural but can serve as opportunities for growth. Surround yourself with positive influences, seek support when needed, and relish the journey toward becoming the best version of yourself.

In the pursuit of wellness, prioritize self-compassion and gratitude, understanding that the commitment to lifelong well-being is a profound investment in your future. As you look ahead, envision a future filled with vitality, purpose, and a deep sense of fulfillment on your continued journey to wellness.

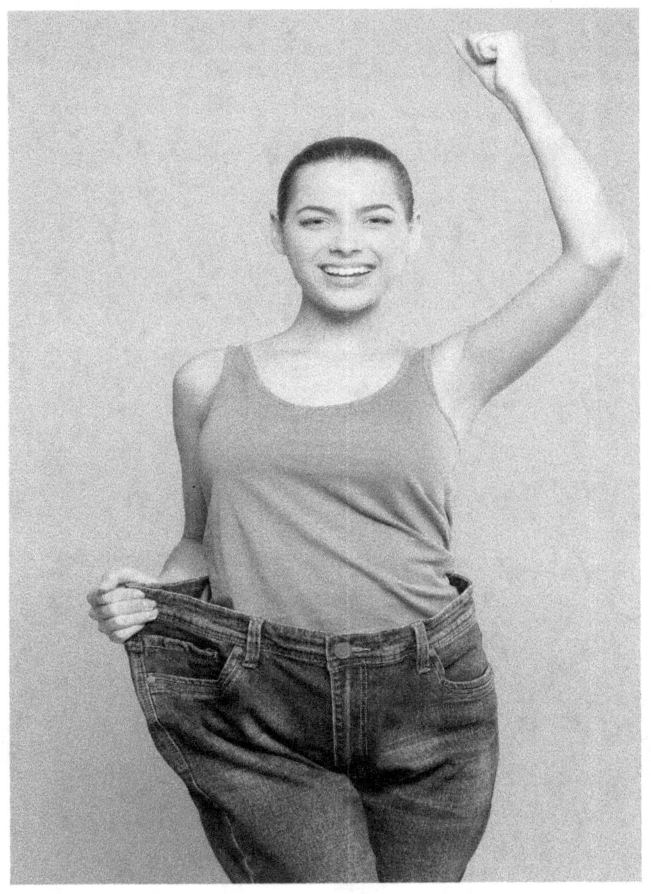